fresh+healthy fresh+healthy fresh+healthy f
resh+healthy fresh+healthy sh+

MW01616146

fresh+healthy fresh+healthy fresh+healthy f
resh+healthy fresh+healthy fresh+healthy fresh+
fresh+healthy fresh+healthy fresh+healthy f
resh+healthy fresh+healthy fresh+healthy fresh+
fresh+healthy fresh+healthy fresh+healthy f
resh+healthy fresh+healthy fresh+healthy fresh+
fresh+healthy fresh+healthy fresh+healthy f
resh+healthy fresh+healthy fresh+healthy fresh+
fresh+healthy fresh+healthy fresh+healthy f
resh+healthy fresh+healthy fresh+healthy fresh+
fresh+healthy fresh+healthy fresh+healthy f
resh+healthy fresh+healthy fresh+healthy fresh+
fresh+healthy fresh+healthy fresh+healthy

SMART
NUTRITION

THE ESSENTIAL VITAMIN, MINERAL & SUPPLEMENT REFERENCE GUIDE

fresh+healthy

Fresh + Healthy Library™

ABOUT THE AUTHOR

Felicia Busch, M.P.H., R.D., F.A.D.A., is president of Felicia Busch & Associates, Inc., a nutrition and health communications company based in St. Paul, Minnesota. She has worked with more than 200 corporate and education clients including national restaurant chains, grocery stores, Fortune 500 companies and international public relations firms to promote good nutrition. Busch is a volunteer national media spokesperson for the American Dietetic Association and has given over 1,800 media interviews on television, radio and in print. She also writes for national magazines, is a contributing author for major consumer books on nutrition, and authored *The New Nutrition: From Antioxidants to Zucchini.*

SMART NUTRITION
The Essential Vitamin, Mineral & Supplement Reference Guide

Printed in 2007.

The nutritional and health information presented in this book is based on an in-depth review of the current scientific literature. It is intended only as an informative resource guide to help you make informed decisions; it is not meant to replace the advice of a physician or to serve as a guide to self-treatment. Always seek competent medical help for any health condition or if there is any question about the appropriateness of a procedure or health recommendation.

Tom Carpenter
Creative Director

Jenya Prosmitsky
Book Design & Production

F+H/Bill Lindner Photography
Main Cover Image

1 2 3 4 5 6 / 11 10 09 08 07
ISBN: 978-1-58159-359-4
© 2002 Fresh + Healthy

Fresh + Healthy
12301 Whitewater Drive
Minnetonka, MN 55343

Contents

Introduction .6

Understanding Nutrition 8

VITAMINS 28

Vitamin A 32

Vitamin C 36

Vitamin D 40

Vitamin E 44

Vitamin K 48

Thiamin or Vitamin B1 52

Riboflavin or Vitamin B2 56

Niacin or Vitamin B3 60

Pyridoxine or Vitamin B6 64

Folic Acid or Vitamin B9 68

Cobalamin or Vitamin B12 72

Pantothenic Acid or Vitamin B5 76

Biotin .80

Choline 84

Inositol 88

MINERALS 90

Boron .94

Calcium 96

Chloride 100

Chromium 102

Copper 106

Fluoride 110

Iodine 114

Iron .118

Magnesium 122

Manganese 126

Molybdenum 130

Phosphorus 132

Potassium 136

Selenium 140

Sodium 144

Zinc .148

SUPPLEMENTS 152

5-Hydroxytryptophan (5-HTP) 156

Acidophilus 158

Alpha-Lipoic Acid (ALA) 160

Arginine 162

Bee Pollen 164

Carnitine 166

Carotenoids 168

Chitosan 170

Chlorophyll 172

Cholestin 174

CoQ-10 176

Creatine 178

Dehydroepiandrosterone (DHEA) 180

Fish Oils—EPA and DHA 182

Flaxseed 184

Fructo-Oligosaccharides (FOS) 186

Gamma Butyrolactone (GBL) 188

Glucosamine 190

Glycerol 192

Kelp 194

L-Tryptophan 196

Lecithin 198

Melatonin 200

PABA 202

Proanthocyanidins 204

Probiotics 206

Psyllium 208

Quercetin 210

Royal Jelly 212

SAM-e 214

Shark Cartilage 216

Soy Isoflavones 218

Spirulina 220

CONDITIONS 222

Alcoholism 226

Allergies, Food 228

Alzheimer's Disease 230

Anemia, Iron Deficiency 232

Arthritis, Osteo 234

Arthritis, Rheumatoid 236

Asthma 238

Cancer 240

Cataracts 242

Depression 244

Diabetes 246

Epilepsy 248

Fibromyalgia 250

Gallstones 252

Heartburn 254

Heart Disease 256

High Blood Pressure 258

High Cholesterol 260

HIV/AIDS 262

Inflammatory Bowel Disease (IBD) 264

Macular Degeneration 266

Menopause 268

Migraine Headaches 270

Multiple Sclerosis (MS) 272

Osteoporosis 274

Premenstrual Syndrome (PMS) 276

Ulcers 278

Index .280

Introduction

UNDERSTAND THE BUILDING BLOCKS OF NUTRITION SO YOU CAN EAT BETTER, LIVE BETTER, FEEL BETTER!

Vitamins, minerals and supplements may not be the most compelling health and wellness topics you consider when creating a healthy lifestyle plan. But without doubt, these building blocks of nutrition lay the foundation upon which your body maintains itself.

Without good nutrition, it's difficult to live life the way it ought to be lived: with energy and enthusiasm.

That's why this special-edition book, exclusive to Fresh + Healthy members, will become an essential resource in your healthy living library.

To start, *Smart Nutrition—The Essential Vitamin, Mineral & Supplement Reference Guide* presents the principles of nutrition in an easy-to-read, easy-to-understand way. You do not have to be a scientist or M.D. to use this book regularly and understand its contents, or to benefit from the messages imparted and put them to use. This truly is everyone's nutrition book!

Then find detailed descriptions of the essential vitamins and minerals you need to consume. True, sometimes the amounts you need are tiny. But every one of these nutritional factors is essential to good metabolism, a properly functioning body, and feeling and looking your best.

Supplements receive extensive coverage too. If you hear about a supplement and think it might be right for you, turn to these pages when it's time to make some decisions. You'll find out what the supplement is, how to buy it, what dangers might be inherent … and how it might (or might not) help you.

And if you have a specific condition you're trying to address, or believe you might be prone to an ailment of some type, you'll want to keep this book available for quick-and-easy reference to those factors. The pages are filled with ideas on how vitamins, minerals

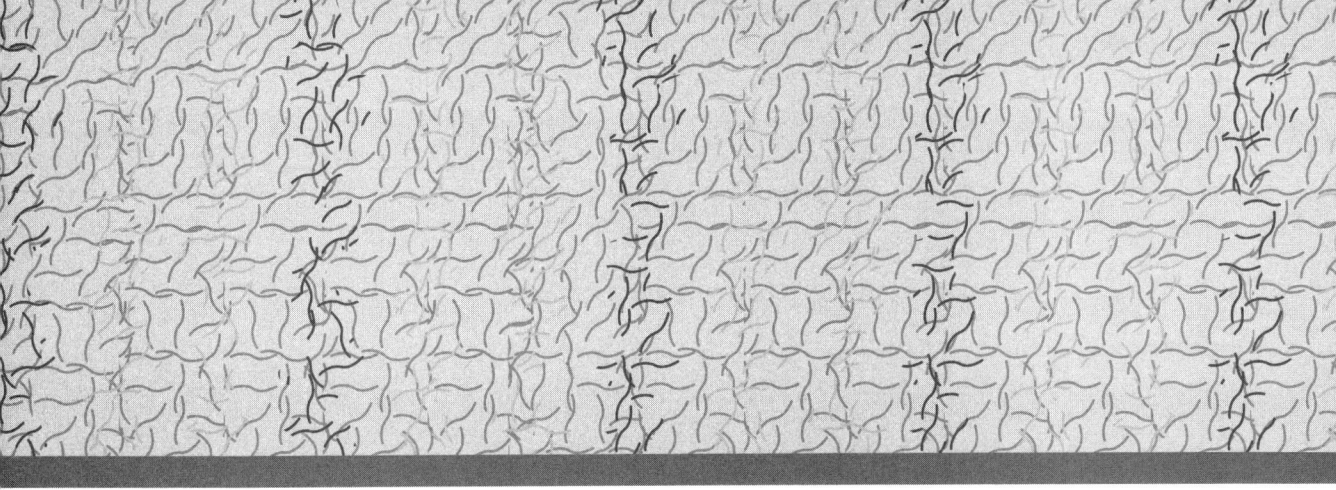

and supplements might be able to address, maybe even prevent, the problem at hand.

This is an important and essential book to have in your Fresh + Healthy Library™. It is a resource that speaks to an important topic—your nutrition—in an understandable way. And it will help you maintain and improve (or maybe create) your own plan for healthy living.

Keep this book on hand, so you can be smart about the nutrition choices and decisions you make. It's all about *Smart Nutrition*. And that has a direct effect on your quality of life.

RECIPE BONUS!

Where space permits, we've included bonus recipes that utilize ingredients that are good sources of the vitamin or mineral being discussed.

fresh+healthy

Understanding Nutrition

You could read seventeen books cover to cover, then spend a hundred hours on the Internet, and still not completely understand the huge topic of "nutrition." Or you could read one succinct, straightforward and logically organized summary and discover—or reaffirm—everything you need to know. That's what you have here. And the message is clear: Strive to get nutrition from food first, supplements second.

Understanding Nutrition

THE NUTRITION CHALLENGE

Food used to be simple. You or your neighbors grew most of it. Labels were not required because it was easy to tell a bushel of corn from a bucket of berries. Everyone prepared food and cooked at home. People ate what was in season and stored extra for the winter months.

In your lifetime, you will eat 80,000 meals, or the equivalent of 70 tons of food and drink. What you eat—and what you avoid eating—can change the odds for or against your long-term health. Every morsel of every meal can help you remain active, vital and strong. Optimal nutrition can help ward off conditions including heart disease, adult-onset diabetes, hypertension, osteoporosis and many other ailments.

Your nutritional needs are unique and different from anyone else's. Yet, all food follows a similar pathway in each of our bodies. Metabolism is responsible for the digestion, absorption, distribution, transformation, storage and excretion of nutrients. Metabolism causes lots of extreme variations in nutrient needs in people born with flaws in their metabolic system. Faulty genes are to blame for nutrition-related disorders that range from lactose intolerance to inherited high blood cholesterol to cystic fibrosis. These types of genetic diseases are called inborn errors of metabolism. Essential enzymes that are missing at birth affect an individual's nutrient needs. Avoiding or restricting particular foods can treat some of these disorders. Other disorders require supplemental nutrients, sometimes in huge amounts, for improvement.

The simple fact that your genetic code is unique means that not all people will benefit equally from improving their eating habits. This explains why some people who "do everything right" develop fatal diseases in their 30s and 40s and others who neglect their health may live to be 100. The challenge of nutrition research today is to identify the genetic traits that need customized dietary planning. One-size-fits-all is no longer an effective approach to nutrition. Of the many environmental factors that can tip the odds in your favor or tilt them against you, food may be the most important. It is fortunately one of the few variables that you can do something about. It's estimated that good nutrition can reduce the incidence of colon cancer by 75 percent, breast cancer by 50 percent and cancer in general by up to 40 percent.

FOOD FIRST

The most recent National Health and Nutrition Examination Survey (NHANES) reports that 80 percent of women and 70 percent of men eat less than two-thirds of the Recommended Dietary Allowance (RDA) for one or more nutrients. At least one-third of the elderly in the United States are nutritionally deficient, and the problem will grow as our population ages.

Why are we eating ourselves into early death and disability? In less than 100 years, we have transformed our society from the farm to the factory and now we're speeding down the information superhighway from our padded office chairs. These changes have impacted both our food and physical activity habits.

Why don't Americans consume enough nutrients from foods? Most of us:
* don't eat enough calories to get adequate vitamin and mineral intakes
* are so inactive that we become overweight despite eating too few calories

- eat a limited variety of food without enough fruits, vegetables and grains
- choose too many processed foods
- take incomplete or haphazardly chosen supplements
- get too few nutrients

Today, grocery store shelves are stuffed with packaged, processed extras. You have to search to find foods that used to be staples. Even "fresh" foods like produce are often several weeks old when they reach your local market.

We're also depending on others to select and prepare our foods. Fast-food drive-through lanes and restaurant eat-in and take-out service are replacing the family dining table. One report from the United States Department of Agriculture's (USDA) Economic Research Service found that meals eaten away from home are much less nutritious than home-prepared foods. Eating out means you get about 25 percent less fiber, calcium and iron than you'd get from foods prepared at home. That's a lot of missed nutrition when you consider that we're now eating almost twice as many meals away from home as we did a decade ago.

OUR DIETS NEED WORK

The U.S. Committee on Dietary Allowances estimates that many Americans consume 30 percent or more of their calories from foods that provide few, if any, vitamins or minerals. A study (see table below) of the dietary sources of nutrients in American adults reports similar results.

CALORIES WITHOUT VITAMINS OR MINERALS

FOOD CATEGORY	PERCENT OF TOTAL CALORIES
cakes, cookies, quick breads and doughnuts	5.5
soft drinks/sodas	4.1
salad dressings/mayonnaise	3.1
margarine	3.0
sugars/syrups/jams	2.8
alcoholic beverages	2.5
potato chips/corn chips/popcorn	2.1
oils	1.0
fruit drinks (not juice)	1.0

Source: Journal of the American Dietetic Association

NUTRITION BASICS

Hidden within foods are hundreds of compounds that take the food-health connection to an exciting new level. Nature planned a clever way to protect its luscious bounty. Smelly sulfur compounds in onion and garlic act as a natural insect repellent. Other plant chemicals, or phytochemicals, protect vegetation from harmful bacteria and viruses. When you eat foods that contain these plant-protecting compounds, they begin to protect you too. They work to halt the forces that zap health in humans—things like cancer, high cholesterol levels and even the aging process.

Animal foods can also play a role in maintaining and promoting health. Their special combination of nutrients provides some of the richest combinations of protein and minerals.

Rely mainly on foods to provide your nutrient needs. Try to eat foods as close to their natural state as possible. A fresh apple is more nutritious than applesauce. Applesauce is a better choice than apple pie—and so on.

WATER

Water is the basis of life. Because your body is nearly two-thirds water, water is the most important nutrient. It's estimated that more than 60 percent of Americans are at least a quart low on water. Do you make the common mistake of waiting until you're thirsty before taking a drink? Thirst isn't an early signal of water needs; it's a warning sign that you're dehydrated and need to drink—and fast. By the time you feel thirsty, you have already lost about 1 percent of your total body water. Subtle signs of dehydration include dry lips, dark-colored urine, muscle or joint soreness, headaches, crankiness and fatigue.

In addition to water, count milk, juice and soup toward your daily fluid intake because of their high water content. Do not include alcohol, coffee, non-herbal tea and soft drinks that contain caffeine; they all have a mild diuretic effect (they make you uri-

nate). In fact, caffeine can hold back water from tissues that need it.

CALORIES

Your body uses energy from the foods you eat to support basic bodily functions and physical activity. This energy comes in the form of calories. Your calorie needs are constantly changing. Infants and teens need the most calories per pound to help meet the demands of sudden growth. Pregnant women also have increased energy needs—especially in the later months of pregnancy.

Unfortunately, calorie needs shrink some with age. But regardless of how many calories you need, your need for important nutrients doesn't shrink. There is no single, easy way to accurately calculate your calorie needs. How much energy you spend in a given task or activity can vary considerably from person to person. A calorie is a unit of energy that you either store or use. You add calories by eating food. You subtract calories by what you do—breathing, walking, talking, exercising and even digesting food. The balance between what you eat and what you do determines your weight and your level of health.

CARBOHYDRATES

There are two types of carbohydrates: simple and complex. Both types are found almost exclusively in plant foods.

Simple carbohydrates are sometimes called simple sugars. Fruit juice and milk products contain the simple carbohydrates fructose and lactose. Sucrose, the most common simple carbohydrate, is found in sweeteners including honey, corn syrup and white sugar. The more important complex carbohydrates are also called starches.

Complex carbohydrates make up a large part of the world food supply such as rice, wheat and corn. Fruit, vegetables and legumes are also complex carbohydrates. Complex carbohydrates are the premium grade of fuel for your body's energy needs because carbohydrates are easily stored in your muscles. These complex carbohydrates break down more slowly than simple sugars and release their available glucose over time.

PROTEIN

Protein is your body's do-it-yourself handyman. Protein helps build and maintain just about everything in your body. From muscles to membranes and blood vessels to bones, protein helps make it and keep it in good repair.

Proteins are made of structural units called amino acids, of which there are 22. Nine of these amino acids you can only get from foods. They are called the essential amino acids. Your body makes the other 13 amino acids as needed. All 22 amino acids link together to form chains. It's like playing Scrabble: You work with the letters you have to build on the base words. Similarly, you need to eat foods containing the essential amino acids to fill each link in the body's amino acid chains to make them complete. Protein is abundant in all animal foods and is found in smaller amounts in most grains and vegetables.

FAT

For years, the message has been that fat is bad and we should all eat less of it. Now researchers are taking a closer look. Maybe fat isn't so bad. After all, it's an essential nutrient needed for good health. Fats are really combinations of many different fatty acids, and each one plays a different role in how your body works. Fat is critical for growth in children, is needed for healthy skin, helps hormone-like substances regulate body processes and is essential for the absorption of fat-soluble vitamins. It is important to note that there is no one best source of fat. Each type of fat (polyunsaturated, monounsaturated and saturated) has its good and bad points. The key is to limit all types of fats.

FIBER

Fiber is the part of a plant that can't be digested by human enzymes. Fiber is found in vegetables, fruits, whole grains and legumes. Because fiber is not digested, it provides no energy or calories. It does provide bulk that helps move waste quickly through your intestinal tract.

There are two main types of fiber: soluble and insoluble. Soluble fiber dissolves in water and forms a gummy substance similar to liquid rubber cement. These gums bind cholesterol and carbohydrates in your intestines, which helps lower blood sugar and blood cholesterol. Insoluble fiber is nature's whisk broom, sweeping out unwanted debris. Insoluble fiber doesn't dissolve in water but acts like an intestinal sponge, soaking up water and expanding the bulk of waste products. That makes your stools softer and easier to move through your intestines. Insoluble fiber reduces the time that waste is in your digestive tract and helps to prevent constipation, hemorrhoids and diverticulosis. Soft bulky stools that move quickly also decrease your chance of developing rectal and colon cancer.

VITAMINS

Vitamins don't have glamorous or exciting names. The first one was named fat-soluble A and the second, water-soluble B. When riboflavin was discovered in 1926, it was found dissolvable in water and was called water-soluble B2. So the original B vitamin became B1. Things really got jumbled when someone figured out that B1 is really two vitamins: thiamin and niacin. Thiamin kept the name B1, and since B2 was already taken, niacin was dubbed B3. And so the story goes. Why isn't there a vitamin B4 or B9?

Overzealous researchers sometimes named a compound a vitamin and then later realized their mistake. It was too messy to continually reassign numbers. Eventually vitamin researchers wised up and started giving names instead of numbers to their discoveries.

Vitamins are chemical compounds containing carbon, which is necessary for growth, health, metabolism and physical well-being. They're found in both plant and animal foods. Some vitamins are essential parts of enzymes—the molecules that help complete chemical reactions. Other vitamins form parts of hormones—substances that promote and protect overall health and reproduction.

Vitamin knowledge is still in its infancy. The first vitamin was discovered less than 100 years ago. Initially, research focused on finding the smallest amount of a nutrient that would prevent common deficiency diseases like scurvy (vitamin C deficiency) and beriberi (thiamin deficiency). Then, as more nutrients were identified, their interactions became important. Today, we're on the threshold of a whole new era, identifying more unique categories of nutrients and learning how they optimize health and thwart disease.

Fat-Soluble Vitamins

Fat-soluble vitamins include vitamins A, D, E and K. They are unique because they are found and stored in fatty tissue. You must eat some fat so these nutrients can be absorbed from foods. Because these vitamins are held in fatty tissue, you don't need to replenish them every day—you can "save them up" over time. However, fat-soluble vitamins have a much greater potential for being toxic, since storage in body fat is almost unlimited.

Water-Soluble Vitamins

The B vitamins plus vitamin C make up the water-soluble nutrients. Unlike their fat-soluble cousins, these can't be stored long-term. B and C vitamins get used up or washed out of your body quickly via urine and sweat. Because they are so fragile, it's easy to lose water-soluble nutrients almost as quickly as you consume them.

MINERALS

Minerals are inorganic chemicals: that is, they are not attached to a carbon atom. They aid biochemical functions necessary for growth, development and overall health. Like vitamins, many minerals are part of enzymes. Minerals help enzymes operate. Different minerals are critical to enzyme systems because they are part of the enzyme itself or because they help the enzyme to work properly. We each need more than 100 milligrams of minerals daily. An adult male has about 5 pounds of minerals stored in his body.

Types of minerals

There are several classifications for dietary minerals, depending on the function they serve and how much you need. They are:

Major minerals—minerals of which you need more than 250 milligrams per day

Electrolytes—minerals that dissolve in water

Trace elements—minerals you need in very tiny amounts, less than 20 milligrams per day

Heavy metals—toxic minerals that can cause harm even in minute amounts, but are still necessary

Colloidal minerals are not a separate or new type of mineral classification. Colloidal refers to the state of matter that is somewhere between a solution and a suspension. Colloidal minerals are tiny mineral particles suspended in a yellowish solution.

(Actually, it's the yellowish color that indicates the presence of these microscopic particles.) Promoters of colloidal minerals claim that the suspension helps improve absorption. However, there is no scientific proof for this theory. The only measurable difference between regular minerals and colloidal minerals is the much higher price tag on colloidal minerals.

Nutrient measures & conversions

Unlike most things we measure, nutrients are weighed using the metric system of grams, milligrams (mg) and micrograms (mcg). These are very tiny measurements; one gram is about the weight of a small paper clip. In fact, your total vitamin and mineral needs for a day would barely add up to an eighth of a teaspoon.

To make things even more complex, some nutrients are measured in more than one way. For example, vitamin A is counted in retinol equivalents (REs), international units (IUs) and beta-carotene equivalencies. In this book, the most common unit of measure is used whenever possible, to make it easier for you to compare food and supplement labels.

CONVERSIONS & EQUIVALENCIES

5 grams = 1 teaspoon

14 grams = ½ ounce = 1 tablespoon = 3 teaspoons

28 grams = 1 ounce = 2 tablespoons

10,000 micrograms = 1,000 milligrams = 1 gram

1 IU of vitamin A = .3 mcg retinol = .6 mcg beta-carotene

1 mg alpha-tocopherol acetate = 1 IU

AMINO ACIDS

Amino acids are the building blocks of protein. Special supplements are not necessary for most people because it's easy to eat foods with plenty of protein. Most amino acid supplements are made from egg protein or animal protein. They can be readily purchased as capsules, tablets and powders. Small amounts of protein-rich foods like milk, meat or eggs can supply significantly more amino acids at a fraction of the cost of supplements.

Regardless of what the supplement ads say, extra protein or amino acids will not increase your muscle mass or improve athletic performance. Because amino acids compete with each other for absorption, too much of one can decrease absorption and utilization of the others.

15

Unsafe aminos

In 1974, the Food and Drug Administration (FDA) removed amino acid supplements from its generally recognized as safe (GRAS) list. Currently, the only approved use for amino acid supplements is medical: Certain health problems like kidney or liver disease may require them as part of intravenous feedings.

ANTIOXIDANTS

Antioxidants are found in foods rich in beta-carotene, vitamin E, vitamin C and selenium. This relatively new category of food chemicals helps protect your body from harmful substances called free radicals, which are unstable oxygen molecules that can cause a lot of damage to your cells.

There are two different types of antioxidants: antioxidant enzymes, which prevent too many free radicals from being produced; and dietary antioxidants, which neutralize free radicals.

Enzymes

Enzymes are proteins that act like biological spark plugs for chemical reactions in your body. Because they are protein molecules, enzymes are inactivated by heat—often at temperatures as low as 115° to 120°F. Your pancreas makes more than enough enzymes for your body. In fact, a single cell contains thousands of enzymes, each with a specific job. Taking enzymes in supplement form is useless because enzymes are almost all broken down into their amino acid building blocks during digestion. Enzymes can't provide any biological benefit when they have been broken down. Only digestive enzymes can survive in the digestive tract and work effectively. Certain digestive enzymes may be taken orally if you are deficient in that particular enzyme (for example, you can take a lactose tablet if you are lactose intolerant). People with chronic pancreas disease might need to take supplemental digestive enzymes.

Ergogenic Aids

The quest for more energy, bigger muscles and less body fat is a popular one. Ergogenic aids sometimes help fuel this search. Ergogenic aids are broadly defined as techniques or substances used for enhancing athletic performance and include food, supplements, drugs, training methods or psychological manipulation. They range from use of reasonable techniques such as carbohydrate loading to illegal and unsafe approaches like anabolic-androgenic steroid use.

Protein is the most popular and enduring ergogenic aid. The notion that massive amounts of protein are necessary during training has evolved from ancient beliefs that great strength could be obtained by eating the raw meat of lions, tigers or other animals that displayed great fighting strength. Although few athletes consume raw meat today,

the idea that "you are what you eat" is still widely promoted by food faddists. The problem is that some athletes go too far with ergogenic aids.

Flavonoids

A class of water-soluble plant pigments, flavonoids are found in a wide range of foods. Flavonoids are broken down into categories, though the issue of how to divide them is not universally agreed upon. Some of the best-known flavonoids include genistein in soy and quercetin in onions. Other flavonoids are hesperidin, rutin and citrus flavonoids.

Hormones

Hormones regulate overall body conditions such as your blood sugar level (insulin hormone) and your metabolic rate (thyroid hormone). Hormones are chemical messengers that target specific tissues or organs. Unlike enzymes, not all hormones are made from protein and they don't start chemical reactions, they just pass messages along. Hormones are highly potent chemical change agents and should not be taken without formal recommendation from a healthcare provider. They are safest when purchased by prescription to ensure purity and quality.

Food Guide

The USDA's Food Guidance System emphasizes variety, proportionality, moderation and activity. MyPyramid (www.MyPyramid.gov) represents specific recommendations for making healthy choices that meet your personal needs. These recommendations are interrelated and are meant to be used together for maximum benefit. The five major food groups—and oils—are symbolized by six bands of the Pyramid. Each food group provides some, but not all, of the nutrients you need. Food in one group can't replace foods in another. No individual food group is more important than another; for good health, you need them all.

MyPyramid.gov
STEPS TO A HEALTHIER YOU

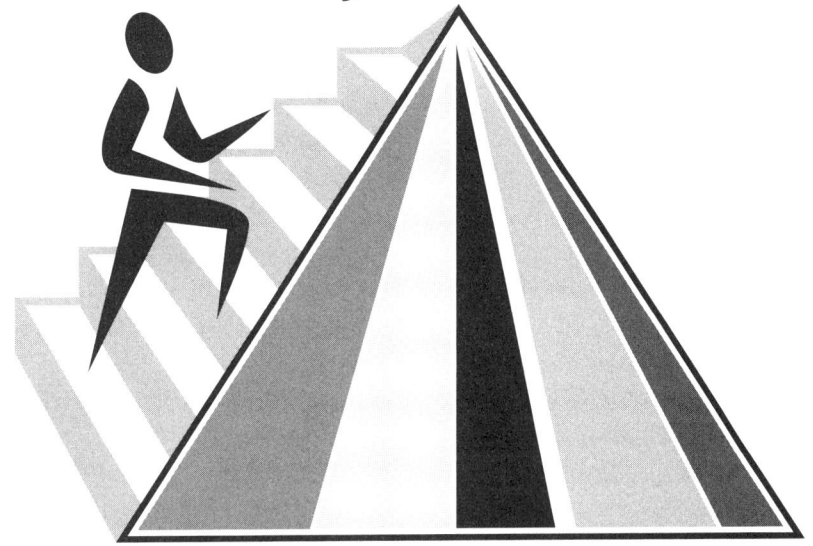

• **Activity** is represented by the steps and the person climbing them, as a reminder of the importance of daily physical activity.

• **Moderation** is represented by the narrowing of each food group from bottom to top. The wider base stands for foods with little or no solid fats or added sugars. These should be selected more often. The narrower top area stands for foods containing more added sugars and solid fats. The more active you are, the more of these foods can fit into your diet.

• **Proportionality** is shown by the different widths of the food group bands. The widths suggest how much food a person should choose from each group. The widths are just a general guide, not exact proportions. Check www.MyPyramid.com to find out how much is right for you.

• **Variety** is symbolized by the Pyramid's six color bands representing the five food groups plus oils. (From left to right, the bands symbolize grains, vegetables, fruits, oils, milk, and meat & beans.) This illustrates that foods from all groups are needed each day for good health.

Following are descriptions and details about each food group. Discover what foods in each group offer the most benefits, and get basic information on good and bad fats.

Grains

These complex carbohydrates provide B-vitamins, minerals and fiber. Steer clear of the more highly processed carbohydrates such as white bread and sugary cereals. Make at least half of your total grains whole grains; they have more vitamins, minerals and fiber than products made from processed white flour. They also hit your bloodstream more slowly, giving you a longer lasting source of fuel.

Vegetables

Naturally low in fat and calories, vegetables are a fantastic source of vitamins and fiber. Deep yellow or orange vegetables like carrots and squash are a great source of vitamin A. Veggies from the cabbage and pepper families (broccoli, brussels sprouts, cabbage, bell peppers) are rich in vitamin C. It's important to eat a variety of vegetables each day and limit starchy vegetables. The variety will help you balance your calorie intake, provide a beneficial variety of nutrients and fiber and, as part of an overall healthy diet, may even help reduce your risk of chronic diseases.

Fruits

Fruits make great snacks or healthy desserts. They're high in carbohydrate energy and potassium, low in sodium and full of vitamins. Strawberries, watermelon and citrus fruits (like oranges and grapefruit) are packed with vitamin C; apricots and other orange-colored fruits have lots of vitamin A; and cantaloupe, mangos and papayas have both vitamins A and C. Avoid canned fruits packed in heavy syrup or juices sweetened with sugar. Also, make the amount of fruit juice you consume less than half your total fruit intake. As with vegetables, eating a variety of fruits will give you an excellent variety of nutrients and fiber and, as part of an overall healthy diet, may even help reduce your risk of chronic diseases.

Milk, Yogurt & Cheese

We've all heard that milk products are rich sources of calcium, but did you know that they're also loaded with protein? A glass of milk or a cup of yogurt has high-quality protein equal to one egg or to an ounce of meat or cheese. Try to choose reduced-fat dairy products whenever possible. A glass of whole milk has the equivalent of 2 teaspoons of butter or 3 tablespoons of sour cream. That bit of added fat would probably be more enjoyable on a baked potato rather than hidden in your milk!

Don't do dairy? If you have lactose intolerance or a dairy allergy, turn to other sources of calcium. Try calcium-fortified beverages, fortified breakfast cereals, sardines or tofu made with calcium.

Meat, Poultry, Fish, Dry Beans, Eggs & Nuts

This group is a major source of protein. Cooked beans are low in fat and high in protein and fiber. Tofu and white beans provide calcium. Almonds are a good source of vitamin E. Beef contains highly

absorbable trace minerals like iron, zinc and manganese. Poultry and seafood provide vitamin B6, and pork is a rich source of thiamine.

Fats, Oils & Sweets

This group includes butter, oils, margarine, sour cream, soda, candy and sweet desserts. Remember, not all fats are created equal. You want to minimize saturated fats found in animal products like meat and dairy, and limit trans fats found in margarine or fried snack foods. Instead, focus on heart-healthy unsaturated fats such as those found in olive oil, nuts, seeds and avocados.

SHORE UP YOUR IMMUNE SYSTEM

At least ten top-selling nutrition books include the word "immunity" in their titles. You might know that immunity is important to your health, but you might wonder just what immunity has to do with the food you eat. In addition to immunizations, the fact is that what you eat can make a big difference in how your body fights off disease and protects itself.

It's hard not to use military adjectives when talking about the human immune system. Its mission is to protect and defend your entire body. There are two main branches of your immune system. The first group is made of defenders that provide general service and fight off everything they encounter to protect you from harm. Your skin, hair, sweat, body oils, saliva and tears are defenders. These immune protectors get physical and set up invasion barriers to protect your internal organs and tissues.

More highly trained, the "special forces" immune protectors launch antibodies that focus on just one type of invader and go for the kill. Together, these specialists are equipped to combat more than 100 billion types of enemies. Specialists have very long memories. If a particular germ has ever attacked you before, the specialist remembers and launches an immediate attack.

Having a decreased level of even a single nutrient can weaken your natural resistance to disease. Sometimes your immune system can get shell-shocked. Your defenders spin out of control and start attacking your own body tissues. A variety of factors help strengthen and protect immunity. Eating a healthful diet that contains a variety of specific nutrients to enhance your immune system is essential. A strong immune system can help you stave off many health problems, in spite of other factors such as family history.

SUPPLEMENTS SECOND

Substantial evidence shows that intakes greater than the RDA (Recommended Dietary Allowance, defined on page 20) of specific vitamins and minerals reduce the risk of particular diseases. A generous intake of the right vitamins and minerals will help you feel and look your best no matter what your age. You might also be able to significantly reduce the risk of chronic, crippling diseases that steal your energy, enjoyment and enthusiasm for life.

But supplements are not magic pills, nor will supplements neutralize the impact of a high-fat, low-fiber diet of overly processed foods. Don't rely on supplements as a nutritional shortcut; you won't come out a winner.

MORE IS NOT ALWAYS BETTER

A megadose of a nutrient is typically any amount greater than 10 times the RDA. At this level, nutrients act differently in your body. Megadoses of some nutrients have significant drug-like effects.

The most frequent side effects from taking too many supplemental nutrients are vague. They include common symptoms such as headache, weakness, fatigue, nausea and vomiting. Often these are the same early symptoms of many other illnesses, including vitamin deficiency. If you notice any early warning signs, be sure to tell your healthcare provider you are taking supplements. It's a good idea to compile a list of all the supplements you're taking and share this with your doctor at every visit.

The facts

With so many myths about supplements, it's important to review the facts:

- Vitamins and minerals don't provide calories or energy.

- All necessary vitamins and minerals can be found in food.

- All vitamins are organic; that is, they contain carbon.

- All minerals are inorganic; that is, they do not contain carbon.

- If you do not consume a particular vitamin or mineral, a deficiency disease will result over time.

TYPE OF TOXICITY

Both one-time overdoses or prolonged over-consumption can cause health impairments. Toxic doses of vitamins and minerals rarely result from eating too much food. Over-supplementation is the culprit. There are three types of vitamin/mineral toxicity:

• **Acute or sudden toxicity** occurs from one very big dose or from several huge doses over a few days. You get sick right away.

• **Chronic toxicity** develops after weeks or months of habitually taking extreme levels of a nutrient. For example, megadoses of vitamin B6 can cause nerve disorders and skin rashes.

There are a variety of scientific standards, none of them perfect, to help sort out how much of a particular nutrient is desirable. Sometimes government and other standards complement each other; often they conflict.

Recommended Dietary Allowances (RDAs), once the gold standard of nutrient recommendations, were designed by the National Academy of Sciences in 1941 for the War Department. They were used as a guide to feeding American soldiers, and the basic concepts haven't changed much in the last 50 years. If you eat close to 100 percent of the RDA for the nutrients listed, you probably have a balanced diet—that is, if you are already a healthy person. For instance, if you consume the RDA for vitamin C (60 mg), you will have a very low risk of scurvy. The RDAs are supposed to tell you how much of each nutrient you need, but even its creators admit that the numbers are not as meaningful as you might hope.

Adequate Intakes (AIs) are the "best guesses" of the experts when not enough science is available to make a formal RDA. Based on a combination of research and observation, they offer a range of intakes that should keep most people healthy.

Daily Values (DVs) and %DVs were invented when the food label was redesigned in 1992. Many people are understandably confused by these new standards. If you are healthy and fit and eat exactly 2,000 calories a day, then the DVs are tailored with you in mind. Since most of us don't follow a daily 2,000-calorie diet, we might need either more or less than 100 percent of the DVs.

Dietary Reference Intakes (DRIs) are the new kids on the block and are promoted as a major leap forward in nutrition science. It's no longer feasible to have a single reference number for each nutrient. DRIs take a broader perspective, examining each nutrient's role in decreasing your risk of developing chronic diseases. It also sets an upper level of intake to protect you from the risk of toxicity. The new goal is more than protection against deficiency; it also aims to lower your risk of major chronic diseases.

The Tolerable Upper Intake Level (UL) is the maximum amount of a nutrient that won't hurt a healthy person. UL is not intended to be a recommended level of intake but a marker for reasonable safety for those who want to "push the envelope." For most nutrients, this number refers to total intake from food, fortified food and nutritional supplements.

Permanent damage may occur with some forms of chronic toxicity. Most people who develop toxic reactions to supplements don't have a clue it's their vitamin or mineral intake that's causing the problem. These people commonly go through an expensive and exhaustive series of tests. Finally, they remember to tell their doctor that they take supplements. If they're lucky, symptoms disappear shortly after stopping supplement consumption.

• **Teratogenic toxicity** refers to harmful changes in a baby's development that occur during pregnancy. Pregnant women risk miscarriage or severe birth defects if they take large amounts of certain supplements, such as vitamin A.

Fortified foods have nutrients added to them during processing. Federal law requires manufacturers to add specific nutrients to certain foods. For example, milk processors add vitamins A and D. Food companies can choose to selectively add almost any nutrient to increase the appeal of a food. For instance, orange juice and rice both come in calcium-fortified versions. Getting nutrients from fortified foods is similar to taking a supplement. There is no guarantee that the form of the nutrient added contains all the known and unknown benefits of eating a real food source.

SUPPLEMENT SAVVY

Have you ever ventured into a casino? Dim lights, smoky air and a rainbow of flashy games entice you to part with your money. You might wonder if the slots are rigged or the dealers crooked, yet the seductive promise of walking away a winner can be difficult to resist. This same image comes to mind when stalking the supplement shelves. The lighting is better and smoking is prohibited, but while you usually don't know what you're getting into, hopes are high for choosing a winner.

Although most people believe otherwise, supplements are one of the most loosely regulated products in America. In 1994, more than two million Americans wrote or called congressional representatives and told them to back off on supplement regulations being proposed by the Dietary Supplement Health and Education Act (DSHEA). Supplement manufacturers misled people into thinking that vitamin supplements would become as regulated as prescription drugs—in other words, limited or difficult to get. The public confusion led to passage of a flimsy set of regulations that fail to provide even minimum standards of safety and truthfulness. Instead of requiring that all types of supplements be proven safe and effective, as is required for foods, drugs and additives, the FDA must wait for proof that a product has caused serious harm or death before it can be pulled from the shelves.

The DSHEA essentially gives dietary supplement manufacturers the freedom to market more products as dietary supplements and provide information about their products' benefits on the label. No license, inspection or quality control is mandated. There are no government specifications for scientific testing of supplements. Each manufacturer can determine what type of testing, if any, will be done. Product manufacturers, not the FDA, also set dosages.

Supplement manufacturers aren't required to completely list the ingredients included in their products. For example, researchers at Cedars-Sinai Bone Center in Los Angeles found that 10 percent of the older people they studied were taking toxic levels of vitamin D. Two of the supplements commonly used by those in the study (which happened to contain some of the highest levels of vitamin D) didn't even list vitamin D as an ingredient.

The United States Pharmacopoeia (USP) sets standards for drug products. They establish standards for individual and combination vitamin and mineral nutritional supplements. These standards detail quality practices for supplement manufacturers. Because the USP is a non-governmental organization, compliance with such standards are voluntary for supplements. However, USP standards for drug products are legally enforceable by the FDA. The USP notation on supplement labels is currently the best way to ensure product quality.

SUPPLEMENT QUALITY INDICATORS

There are several key measures that are important in making sure that vitamin and mineral tablets and capsules do the job you expect them to do. The following quality indicators are based on USP laboratory testing standards:

• **Disintegration** measures how fast a tablet or capsule breaks into small pieces. Smaller sized pieces allow the ingredients to dissolve more easily. If a tablet or capsule does not break down within a certain amount of time, it may pass through your body without being absorbed. Water-soluble vitamins should disintegrate in less than 45 minutes (uncoated) or in less than 60 minutes (coated).

• **Dissolution** gauges how fast and how much of a vitamin or mineral dissolves in a fluid that is similar to your digestive tract. USP standards track pyridoxine (vitamin B6) when testing multivitamins. Their standards require that 75 percent be dissolved within 60 minutes.

• **Strength** is the amount of a specific vitamin or mineral substance in each tablet or capsule. To meet USP product quality standards, the amount present must be within a narrow range of the amount declared on the label.

• **Purity** is controlled by USP standards that set a range for acceptable impurities that can result from contamination or degradation of the product during processing or storage.

• **Expiration** dates must be imprinted on the package. When the date is past due, the nutrient ingredients in a bottle or package of supplements may no longer meet USP standards of purity, strength and/or quality.

It's been widely reported that you can test your own supplements at home for disintegration. However, home experiments using water or vinegar don't come close to copying the conditions in your stomach or at a laboratory.

THE CLAIM GAME

The DSHEA allows dietary supplements to carry "structure or function" claims, but it does not allow statements by manufacturers implying that their products can treat, diagnose, cure or prevent disease. All structure or function claims must be based on scientific studies that have proven the health benefits of using supplements. However, the supplement manufacturer or its advertising agency defines the term "scientific." Thumb through magazine ads for supplements and you'll see that almost anything counts as scientific in the minds of the companies that market these products.

Benefit claims have always been a controversial feature of dietary supplement labeling, and manufacturers rely on those claims to sell products. Can you trust them? The DSHEA and previous food-labeling laws allow supplement manufacturers to use three types of claims. Nutrient-content claims and health claims follow rules similar to those required for food products. Nutrition support claims, which include "structure-function claims," are unique to supplement products. As with food products, nutrient levels required for any claims are based on DV, and not RDA (see definitions, page 20).

Structure-Function Claims

Structure-function claims refer to the supplement's effect on the body's structure or function, including its overall effect on a person's well-being. Examples of structure-function claims are:

• calcium builds strong bones.
• antioxidants maintain cell integrity.
• fiber maintains bowel regularity.

Manufacturers can use structure-function claims without FDA authorization. Structure-function claims are easy on the label because they must be accompanied with this disclaimer: "This statement has not been evaluated by the Food and Drug Administration. This product is not intended to diagnose, treat, cure or prevent any disease."

Nutrient-Content Claims

Nutrient-content claims describe the level of a nutrient in a food or dietary supplement. For example, a supplement containing at least 200 milligrams of calcium per serving could carry the claim "high in calcium" since it provides at least 20% of the DV for calcium. A supplement with at least 12 milligrams per serving of vitamin C could state on its label, "Excellent source of vitamin C."

Health Claims

Health claims indicate a link between a food or substance and a disease or health-related condition. The FDA preauthorizes these claims based on a review of the scientific evidence or authoritative statements from certain scientific bodies, such as the National Academy of Sciences, that show or describe a well-established diet-to-health link. As of this writing, a few of the approved claims include:

* a link between folic acid and a decreased risk of neural tube defect-affected pregnancy (if the supplement contains sufficient amounts of folic acid).

* a link between calcium and a lower risk of osteoporosis (if the supplement contains sufficient amounts of calcium).

* a link between psyllium seed husk (as part of a diet low in cholesterol and saturated fat) and a lower risk of coronary heart disease (if the supplement contains sufficient amounts of psyllium seed husk).

Examples of prohibited claims for a dietary supplement include "protects against cancer," "treats hot flashes," and "reduces nausea associated with chemotherapy." If you find dietary supplements whose labels state or imply that the product can help diagnose, treat, cure or prevent a disease (for example, "cures cancer" or "treats arthritis"), remember that the product is being marketed illegally as a drug and has not been evaluated for safety or effectiveness.

Nutrition Support Claims

Nutrition support claims describe a link between a nutrient and the deficiency disease that can result if the nutrient is lacking in the diet. For example, an

ANATOMY OF THE NEW REQUIREMENTS FOR DIETARY SUPPLEMENT LABELS

Information required on supplement labels includes:

- Statement of identity (for example, "vitamin C").
- Net quantity of contents (for example, "100 capsules").
- Optional structure-function claim must include the warning "This statement has not been evaluated by the Food and Drug Administration. This product is not intended to diagnose, treat, cure or prevent any disease."
- Directions for use (for example, "Take one capsule daily").
- Supplement facts panel (serving size, amount and active ingredient).
- Other ingredients in descending order of predominance and by common name or proprietary blend.
- Name and place of business of manufacturer, packer or distributor. This is the address you would use to obtain more product information.

Source: Adapted from the FDA Consumer

iron supplement label could state: "iron prevents anemia." When these types of claims are used, the label must mention the prevalence of the nutrient-deficiency disease in the United States.

In an effort to correct these problems, the FDA is trying to update the DSHEA. By clarifying for manufacturers what types of claims can and cannot be made on a dietary supplement label, newer legislation may help consumers make more informed and wiser choices.

REGULATING THE CLAIMS

The Federal Trade Commission (FTC), not the FDA, regulates claims made in the advertising of dietary supplements. In recent years, the FTC has taken a number of enforcement actions against companies whose advertisements contained false and misleading information. Erroneous claims that chromium picolinate was a treatment for weight loss and high blood cholesterol were removed. One action targeted ads for an ephedrine alkaloid supplement because they understated the degree of the product's risk and featured a man falsely described as a doctor.

According to many professional groups, including the American Dietetic Association (ADA), consumer perception of supplement claims should also be part of the decision-making process. For instance, just what does "strengthen immunity" mean to the average supplement shopper? Preliminary research by the FDA shows that current health claims lead consumers to believe that products are likely to have positive health effects well beyond those promoted on the label.

Ads for supplements have powerful messages that play on consumers' fears and exploit the desire to find an easy and "natural" solution to eating right. The FDA has little control over dietary supplements. This means that consumers have the responsibility for checking the safety of dietary supplements and determining the truthfulness of any label claims.

The FTC gives consumers a little assistance in evaluating advertising claims by releasing a business guide for the dietary supplement industry. This guide spells out that anyone who "participates directly or indirectly in the marketing of dietary supplements has an obligation to make sure that claims are presented truthfully and to check the adequacy of the support." According to the FTC, the amount and type of support will depend on a variety of factors. These factors include consumers' expectations of what a claim means, the specific claim being made, how claims are presented in the context of the entire ad and how statements are qualified.

In evaluating the adequacy of support for a claim, the FTC expects to consult with experts in a wide variety of fields, including those with a background in botanical and traditional medicines. The FTC's definition of dietary supplements includes vitamins, minerals, herbal products, hormones and amino acids.

SUPPLEMENT PROFITEERS

It's not just the claims that are fraudulent; it's also the prices. In one case, the U.S. Department of Justice won its largest case ever, with fines of $725 million, against several giant foreign drug and chemical companies, for engaging in a worldwide conspiracy to raise and fix the prices of vitamins and other supplements. It's estimated that the inflated prices in effect since January 1990 affected more than $5 billion of common products ranging from vitamins and enriched foods including milk, cereal and pet foods.

The U.S. market for vitamins and supplements is projected to be worth between $11 and $20 billion. The editor of the *Nutrition Business Journal* estimates that mainstream physicians directly sold about $120 million worth of supplements to their patients last year. Chiropractors, homeopaths, naturopaths and other alternative practitioners sold an additional $680 million in supplements from their offices.

For years, the federal government has frowned upon doctors sending blood and urine samples to their own labs for analysis. The concern is that extra tests will be ordered to add profits to the balance sheet. The American Medical Association Code of Medical Ethics says physicians should not let their wallets influence what they prescribe. Would your doctors sell supplements to you if doing so would double their income from your office visits?

Personal selling creates the lion's share of wealth in the supplement industry. Pyramid selling programs like Amway, Rexall and Shaklee allow anyone to sell supplements. These salespeople benefit personally when you take their advice, as does the eager health food store employee who works on commission. If you've ever been asked to sell supplements, you are probably aware that more time and energy goes into training you to be a super-salesperson than knowing much about what you sell.

What should you spend?

If you are spending more than $10 a month on vitamin/mineral supplements, you're paying too much.

PROTECTING YOUR INVESTMENT

Here's how to get the most for your supplement money:

* Choose only vitamin/mineral supplements designated as meeting USP guidelines to ensure you are getting a quality product that will deliver what's listed on the label.
* Don't pay extra for "natural" supplements—they all work the same. Minerals are always natural since they can't be made from other substances. Vitamins present in food and plants are considered natural vitamins. Vitamins created in a laboratory are synthetic. There is no difference in most vitamin molecules whether they are synthetic or natural. Synthetic vitamins are usually less expensive, their potency can be better controlled and they may be purer or less contaminated with pesticides and fertilizers. On the other hand, natural vitamins may, by default, include other food components that are beneficial to health. One notable exception to this rule is vitamin E. The natural form of vitamin E (alpha-tocopherol) varies slightly from the synthetic versions (beta-, delta- and gamma-tocopherol), and the nutrient is more effective in the natural form.
* Generics can be a good deal. National retailers like K-Mart, Target and WalMart purchase supplements that are often identical to the higher priced name brands. Compare the labels.
* High potency claims on a supplement label will cost you more. Since "high potency" is not legally defined, anyone can slap the term on a supplement label. It means nothing.
* Supplements work best when taken in several small doses spread throughout the day. That's because you can absorb more of a nutrient when your system isn't overloaded. When a high concentration of a nutrient enters your bloodstream, your kidneys work to quickly get rid of the excess. Taking a one-shot supplement isn't ideal, but it is convenient. Time-released supplements don't offer much of an advantage. Since vitamins and minerals are absorbed at different places in the gastrointestinal tract, it's highly unlikely that a time-released tablet will deliver each nutrient at the optimal time and place for absorption.
* Vitamin sprays and patches are sold in some parts of the United States and Canada. Contrary to their marketing literature, it has not been proven that you can absorb more nutrients because they have been applied to your skin or sprayed inside your mouth.
* Take your multivitamin/mineral supplements with food and water. You need fat and water to maximize nutrient absorption.
* Avoid frills and extras such as glandular products, hormones and amino acids. All of these add-ons can increase the cost of a supplement without a proven benefit. Supplements that include such products

often do not completely label or disclose the total amounts of nutrients they contain, and may result in potentially toxic doses.

• Check expiration dates. Never purchase supplements past their expiration dates—no matter how cheap they are. In fact, if a product is within 6 months of expiring, you can be sure it's lost some of its stability and potency.

If money is scarce, spend it on produce instead of supplements. Eating a variety of wholesome foods has a greater benefit than taking supplements to correct poor nutritional status.

Storing supplements

Never store supplements anywhere in your bathroom. The heat and moisture variations may change the action of the vitamin or speed deterioration. Store supplements tightly capped and safely out of the reach of young children. Most supplements do best in a cool, dry place away from direct sunlight. A high shelf in the kitchen, away from the oven or stove, is usually a good choice.

EXPERT EVALUATION

If you have a chronic disease, complicated eating preferences or just like the idea of checking out your food intake, it's critical to find a reputable professional to help guide you. As with all trades or professions, there is a range of competencies among those who practice. Team up with someone who has a strong academic and practical background in food, nutrition and health. They should be able to personalize suggestions and offer strategies right for you.

Memorizing the chemical structures of vitamins or digestive pathways doesn't make someone a nutrition expert. Many health professionals, including doctors and nurses, learn the biology of nutrition. Most don't have a clue how to translate that into what to eat in order to attain optimal health. The endorsement of special diets or nutrition products by people with a string of initials after their name should make you skeptical. Nutrition professionals shouldn't be endorsing specific products. Don't hand over your money to hucksters and celebrities. They may be great salespeople, but they are not usually great nutrition advisors.

WHO'S WHO IN NUTRITION

It is important to understand what the various titles really mean when it comes to evaluating nutritional professionals and their credentials. Here's a rundown.

REGISTERED DIETITIAN (RD)

No doubt about it, RDs are the nutrition experts in the United States. No other group of individuals has the integrated training in the art and science of food and nutrition. An RD separates fact from fiction. He or she can explain the latest scientific findings in an easy-to-understand way. An RD gives you personal attention and helps you create an eating plan and nutrition program that is uniquely yours.

RDs must complete a bachelor's or master's degree in nutrition, dietetics, public health, biochemistry, medicine or other nutrition specialty from an accredited college or university. As part of (or in addition to) this schooling, RDs must perform a rigorous, supervised internship. When the learning and practice are completed, there's a national exam to pass, and continuing professional education is mandatory. Only 23 states require licensing of dietitians and nutritionists. The only credible national credential for a nutrition expert is the RD.

Nutritionist

If you decide to see a nutritionist, be sure to ask what other credentials he or she has. Anyone can claim the title of nutritionist, and there are no credentials, knowledge, training or ethics required. The term nutritionist is not federally regulated and neither are its practitioners. However, the public health service and the Special Supplemental Nutrition Program for Women, Infants and Children (WIC) still use the term nutritionist in job descriptions that dietitians normally fill.

Certified Nutritional Consultant (CNC)

The trademark designation CNC after a Nutritional Consultant's name indicates they are a member of the American Association of Nutritional Consultants (AANC). Membership or certified membership in this association doesn't mean that someone is qualified to practice nutrition. "Membership in AANC and its predecessors has been open to anyone," says Dr. Stephen Barrett, a leading authority on medical fraud. To prove that fact, years ago, Victor Herbert, M.D., J.D., a prominent nutrition scientist, obtained an AANC "professional membership" for his dog by sending $50 plus the name and address of his pet. Today's fees are higher ($150) and members are required to take an open-book, at-home exam. According to the AANC's Web site, "We realize that after looking over the tests, the candidate may feel that he or she needs to review one or more of the subjects. Therefore, we include with the examination a list of recommended textbooks. The textbooks recommended are those which will assist the candidate in successfully completing these specific portions of the examination the candidate finds troubling."

Vitamins

The list of vitamins you need is finite, but your need for vitamins never ends. It is important to understand what each vitamin is and what it does for you, as well as how much you should get. Maybe more important, you need to know how to get that vitamin in a natural way so that your body can make use of it. Here is all of that information, and more, for the vitamins that sustain life itself.

How to Use This Chapter

Each vitamin is described in a variety of ways:

What Is It?
A brief description of the nutrient.

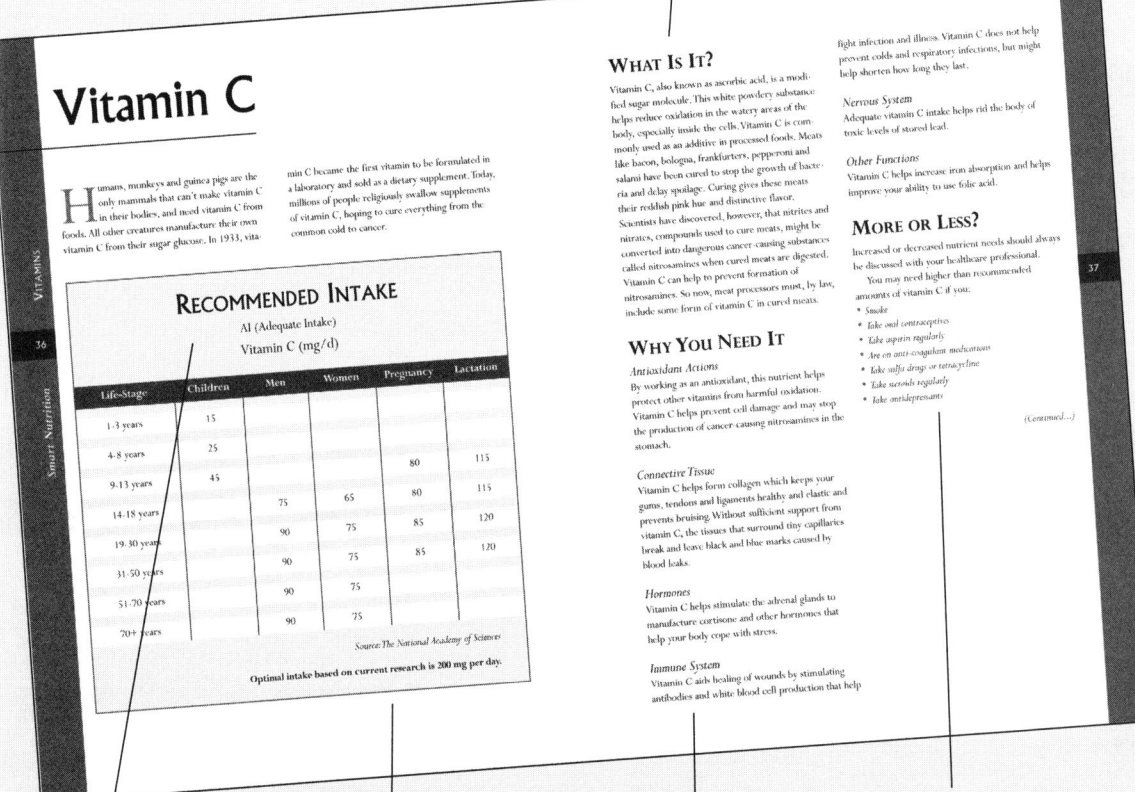

Recommended Intake
These are the highest current recommendations based on federal guidelines.

Optimal Intake
These levels might be higher than the current RDA or DV (defined on page 20). Optimal intake amounts are based on the analysis of scientific studies, review papers and interviews with leading experts.

Why You Need It
This section summarizes the main functions of the nutrient based on the following classifications:

- Antioxidant Actions
- Bones & Teeth
- Energy Production
- Hormonal Balance
- Immune System
- Metabolism
- Nervous System & Brain
- Skin & Hair
- Other Functions

More or Less?
Individual differences such as lifestyle, chronic disease status and other factors can increase or decrease your need for a particular nutrient. Use this section as a starting point to discuss individual needs with your healthcare provider. Never take more or less than the recommended or optimal amounts of any nutrient without professional guidance.

Best Natural Food Sources

These are foods that provide at least 25 percent of the RDA in just one serving. Liver or organ meats were purposely omitted from these lists, even though they might be excellent vitamin or mineral sources, because an animal's liver is also its toxic waste dump. The risk of harm from consuming toxic substances far outweighs the benefit of concentrated nutrients.

Fortified Foods

Instead of relying on fortified foods, eat foods naturally high in nutrients. Nature's combination of nutrients helps your body absorb and utilize vitamins and minerals. A product fortified with one or more nutrients will not provide the complex package of compounds found in food. Eating fortified foods is a second-rate choice.

Think Twice!

Warning notices for potential interactions are noted here.

Did You Know?

With so many myths and miscommunications about the value and use of supplements, it's easy to become confused. Common questions or concerns are addressed here to help you separate fact from fiction.

Kitchen Connections

This information will help you learn to make smart food choices and preserve nutrients in foods that you store and prepare at home.

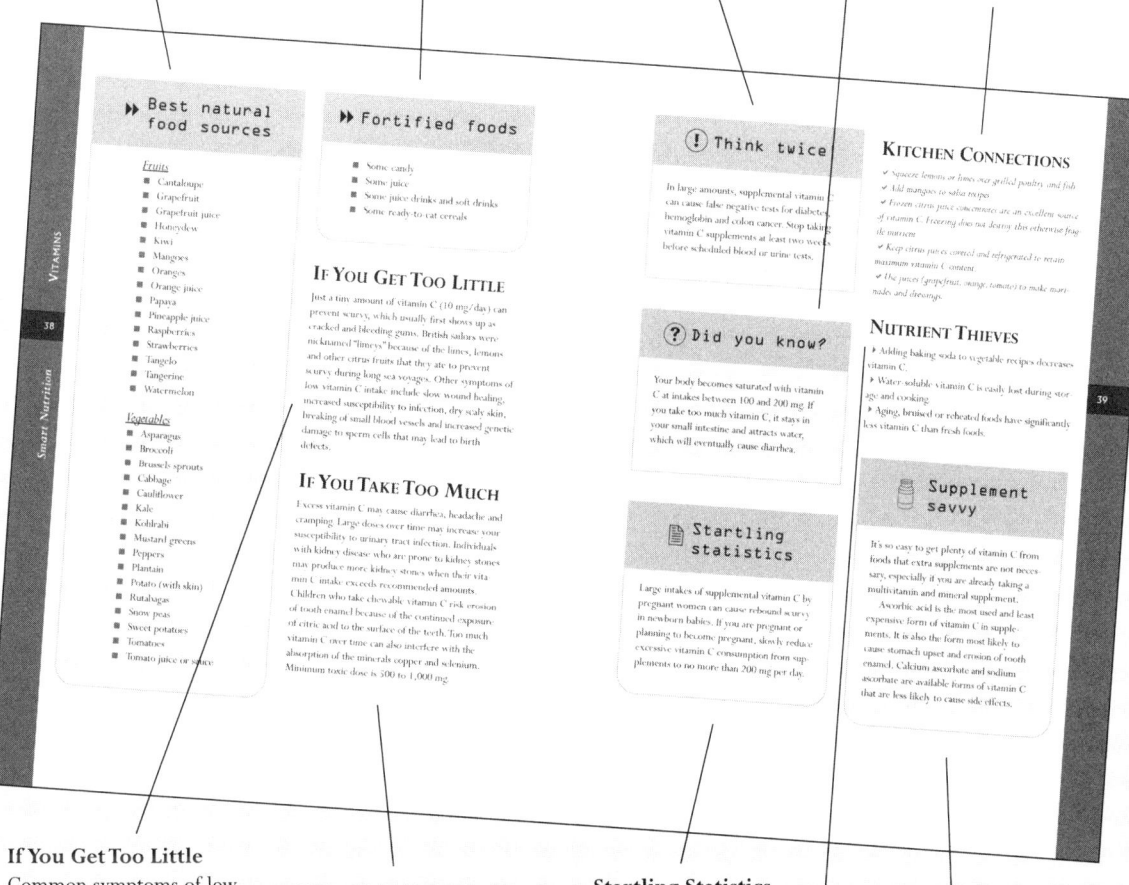

If You Get Too Little

Common symptoms of low intakes are described, as are the full-blown symptoms of a deficiency disease.

If You Take Too Much

The key word here is *take*. It's almost impossible to get too much of a nutrient from foods. Misuse of supplements is almost always the reason for the side effects listed. The minimum toxic dose is given, when known. This is the smallest amount of a nutrient that can cause side effects ranging from annoying to life threatening.

Startling Statistics

These will help you put things into perspective.

Supplement Savvy

If you must take a supplement, here are the facts to help you make an informed choice.

Nutrient Thieves

This information will help you identify those things that destroy or rob your foods of nutrients. You will also learn how to prevent nutrient loss.

Vitamin A

The first vitamin discovered, vitamin A, is evident in the natural coloring of foods: the brilliant red in a pepper, the deep orange in a carrot or the golden yellow hues in squash. Sometimes the color of vitamin A is masked by a deep green color, so it can be found in some leafy green vegetables too.

WHAT IS IT?

Vitamin A is a family of fat-soluble nutrient compounds called retinoids that are stored in your liver. Vitamin A is found in two forms: preformed vitamin A, also called retinol, is found only in animal foods. Provitamin A, or beta-carotene, is stored in plant

RECOMMENDED INTAKE

RDA (Recommended Dietary Allowance)

Vitamin A (IU/d)

Life-Stage	Children	Men	Women	Pregnancy	Lactation
1-3 years	300				
4-8 years	400				
9-13 years	600			750	1200
14-18 years		900	700	750	1200
19-30 years		900	700	770	1300
31-50 years		900	700	770	1300
51-70 years		900	700		
70+ years		900	700		

Source: The National Academy of Sciences

foods (see carotenes). Vitamin A is best absorbed in the presence of some dietary fat.

WHY YOU NEED IT

Bones & Teeth

Growth and development of teeth and bones depend on an adequate supply of vitamin A, especially during infancy and the years of rapid growth.

Immune System

Vitamin A helps stimulate the immune system to line your air passages and digestive tract with protective cells that resist infection. Optimal intakes of vitamin A may strengthen the immune system and fend off certain cancers. Vitamin A helps protect body surfaces designed to keep infection and disease out. These special surfaces include your skin and the moist lining of your mouth, throat and digestive tract. Vitamin A's influence on immunity may be one of the ways it helps prevent the initiation or growth of cancer cells.

Skin & Hair

Vitamin A is essential for normal growth and healthy development of all body tissues and helps maintain the protective layers of your skin, especially the eyes.

Other

Vitamin A combines with a special protein in your eye to improve night vision and aid color perception. Night blindness is the slow recovery of vision after bright flashes of light in the dark. Bright light bleaches eye pigments that are normally regenerated by retinal in the eye.

MORE OR LESS?

Increased or decreased nutrient needs should always be discussed with your healthcare professional.

You may need higher than recommended amounts of vitamin A if you have:

- Cystic fibrosis
- Diabetes
- Gout
- Intestinal disease with diarrhea
- Liver disease
- Kidney disease
- Pancreatic disease

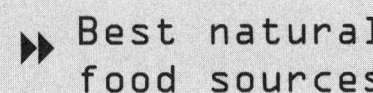

▶▶ Best natural food sources

- Apricots
- Cantaloupe
- Carrots
- Kale
- Mangoes
- Peppers
- Pumpkin
- Spinach
- Squash
- Sweet potatoes
- Turnip greens

▶▶ Fortified foods

- Low-fat and skim milk
- Margarine
- Some ready-to-eat cereals

IF YOU GET TOO LITTLE

Signs of vitamin A deficiency include poor night vision, decreased resistance to infection, extremely dry skin and dull hair. In children, mild vitamin A deficiency may increase a child's risk for respiratory infection and decrease growth rate, bone development and the likelihood of survival from serious illness. Xerophthalmia is the deficiency disease that results from too little vitamin A. When the mucous (moisture) membranes in the eye dry out, small particles of dirt may settle there. Bacteria can enter the vulnerable eye through the scratches caused by these dirt particles. White blood cells, which help fight infection, start attacking bacteria in the scratches and cause lesions. As these lesions grow, blindness can result.

IF YOU TAKE TOO MUCH

Toxic levels of vitamin A may cause blurred vision, diarrhea, headaches, irritability, muscle weakness, scaling or peeling of skin and vomiting. In growing children, excess vitamin A can cause premature bone closures that result in deformities. Too much vitamin A is also known to cause stunted growth in children. During pregnancy, vitamin A toxicity causes a variety of serious birth defects. Many prescription and over-the-counter acne medications contain high levels of vitamin A (as retinoic acid) that should be avoided by women who may become pregnant. The minimum toxic dose of vitamin A is 6,500 IU per day.

! Think twice!

If you are a heavy drinker, high levels of vitamin A or beta-carotene can damage your liver.

Don't take additional vitamin A supplements (other than prescribed prenatal vitamins) if you are pregnant. Too much vitamin A may cause serious birth defects.

? Did you know?

People who eat at restaurants at least once a week consume less vitamin A than people who eat at home. That's because most restaurant meals lack deep yellow and orange vegetables rich in vitamin A. If you eat out frequently, be sure to eat foods rich in vitamin A at home and for snacks.

The American Academy of Pediatrics recommends that all children 6 to 24 months of age hospitalized with measles and all hospitalized children over 6 months with a poor nutrition history receive vitamin A supplementation. That's because enough American children are at risk for mild vitamin A deficiency that supplementation may significantly improve their recovery.

Startling statistics

Polar bear liver is the only animal source of vitamin A known to cause toxic or even fatal effects. That's because polar bear liver has up to 40,000 times the RDA of vitamin A.

KITCHEN CONNECTIONS

✔ *Remember: The more intense the color of the fruit or vegetable, the higher the vitamin A content. Look for deep yellow and orange.*

✔ *Increase your intake by eating these foods rich in vitamin A:*

• *Add spinach leaves to salads and sandwiches.*

• *Add pureed carrots to soup.*

• *Add a sweet potato to the white potatoes in your favorite mashed potato recipe.*

• *Add grated carrots to meatloaf.*

• *Top hot or cold cereal with dried apricot bits.*

• *Try carrot-based juices.*

• *Add fresh peppers to salads and pasta dishes.*

NUTRIENT THIEVES

▶ Exposure to light, heat or air can reduce levels of vitamin A in foods.

▶ Mineral oil and laxative use can dramatically decrease available fat-soluble vitamins, including vitamin A.

Supplement savvy

Do not take individual supplements of vitamin A; the potential risks are too great.

Vitamin C

Humans, monkeys and guinea pigs are the only mammals that can't make vitamin C in their bodies, and need vitamin C from foods. All other creatures manufacture their own vitamin C from their sugar glucose. In 1933, vita-min C became the first vitamin to be formulated in a laboratory and sold as a dietary supplement. Today, millions of people religiously swallow supplements of vitamin C, hoping to cure everything from the common cold to cancer.

RECOMMENDED INTAKE

AI (Adequate Intake)

Vitamin C (mg/d)

Life-Stage	Children	Men	Women	Pregnancy	Lactation
1-3 years	15				
4-8 years	25				
9-13 years	45			80	115
14-18 years		75	65	80	115
19-30 years		90	75	85	120
31-50 years		90	75	85	120
51-70 years		90	75		
70+ years		90	75		

Source: The National Academy of Sciences

Optimal intake based on current research is 200 mg per day.

WHAT IS IT?

Vitamin C, also known as ascorbic acid, is a modified sugar molecule. This white powdery substance helps reduce oxidation in the watery areas of the body, especially inside the cells. Vitamin C is commonly used as an additive in processed foods. Meats like bacon, bologna, frankfurters, pepperoni and salami have been cured to stop the growth of bacteria and delay spoilage. Curing gives these meats their reddish pink hue and distinctive flavor. Scientists have discovered, however, that nitrites and nitrates, compounds used to cure meats, might be converted into dangerous cancer-causing substances called nitrosamines when cured meats are digested. Vitamin C can help to prevent formation of nitrosamines. So now, meat processors must, by law, include some form of vitamin C in cured meats.

WHY YOU NEED IT

Antioxidant Actions
By working as an antioxidant, this nutrient helps protect other vitamins from harmful oxidation. Vitamin C helps prevent cell damage and may stop the production of cancer-causing nitrosamines in the stomach.

Connective Tissue
Vitamin C helps form collagen which keeps your gums, tendons and ligaments healthy and elastic and prevents bruising. Without sufficient support from vitamin C, the tissues that surround tiny capillaries break and leave black and blue marks caused by blood leaks.

Hormones
Vitamin C helps stimulate the adrenal glands to manufacture cortisone and other hormones that help your body cope with stress.

Immune System
Vitamin C aids healing of wounds by stimulating antibodies and white blood cell production that help fight infection and illness. Vitamin C does not help prevent colds and respiratory infections, but might help shorten how long they last.

Nervous System
Adequate vitamin C intake helps rid the body of toxic levels of stored lead.

Other Functions
Vitamin C helps increase iron absorption and helps improve your ability to use folic acid.

MORE OR LESS?

Increased or decreased nutrient needs should always be discussed with your healthcare professional.

You may need higher than recommended amounts of vitamin C if you:
* Smoke
* Take oral contraceptives
* Take aspirin regularly
* Are on anti-coagulant medications
* Take sulfa drugs or tetracycline
* Take steroids regularly
* Take antidepressants

(Continued...)

▶▶ Best natural food sources

Fruits
- Cantaloupe
- Grapefruit
- Grapefruit juice
- Honeydew
- Kiwi
- Mangoes
- Oranges
- Orange juice
- Papaya
- Pineapple juice
- Raspberries
- Strawberries
- Tangelo
- Tangerine
- Watermelon

Vegetables
- Asparagus
- Broccoli
- Brussels sprouts
- Cabbage
- Cauliflower
- Kale
- Kohlrabi
- Mustard greens
- Peppers
- Plantain
- Potato (with skin)
- Rutabagas
- Snow peas
- Sweet potatoes
- Tomatoes
- Tomato juice or sauce

▶▶ Fortified foods

- Some candy
- Some juice
- Some juice drinks and soft drinks
- Some ready-to-eat cereals

IF YOU GET TOO LITTLE

Just a tiny amount of vitamin C (10 mg/day) can prevent scurvy, which usually first shows up as cracked and bleeding gums. British sailors were nicknamed "limeys" because of the limes, lemons and other citrus fruits that they ate to prevent scurvy during long sea voyages. Other symptoms of low vitamin C intake include slow wound healing, increased susceptibility to infection, dry scaly skin, breaking of small blood vessels and increased genetic damage to sperm cells that may lead to birth defects.

IF YOU TAKE TOO MUCH

Excess vitamin C may cause diarrhea, headache and cramping. Large doses over time may increase your susceptibility to urinary tract infection. Individuals with kidney disease who are prone to kidney stones may produce more kidney stones when their vitamin C intake exceeds recommended amounts. Children who take chewable vitamin C risk erosion of tooth enamel because of the continued exposure of citric acid to the surface of the teeth. Too much vitamin C over time can also interfere with the absorption of the minerals copper and selenium. Minimum toxic dose is 500 to 1,000 mg.

! Think twice!

In large amounts, supplemental vitamin C can cause false negative tests for diabetes, hemoglobin and colon cancer. Stop taking vitamin C supplements at least two weeks before scheduled blood or urine tests.

? Did you know?

Your body becomes saturated with vitamin C at intakes between 100 and 200 mg. If you take too much vitamin C, it stays in your small intestine and attracts water, which will eventually cause diarrhea.

Startling statistics

Large intakes of supplemental vitamin C by pregnant women can cause rebound scurvy in newborn babies. If you are pregnant or planning to become pregnant, slowly reduce excessive vitamin C consumption from supplements to no more than 200 mg per day.

KITCHEN CONNECTIONS

- ✔ *Squeeze lemons or limes over grilled poultry and fish.*
- ✔ *Add mangoes to salsa recipes.*
- ✔ *Frozen citrus juice concentrates are an excellent source of vitamin C. Freezing does not destroy this otherwise fragile nutrient.*
- ✔ *Keep citrus juices covered and refrigerated to retain maximum vitamin C content.*
- ✔ *Use juices (grapefruit, orange, tomato) to make marinades and dressings.*

NUTRIENT THIEVES

- ▸ Adding baking soda to vegetable recipes decreases vitamin C.
- ▸ Water-soluble vitamin C is easily lost during storage and cooking.
- ▸ Aging, bruised or reheated foods have significantly less vitamin C than fresh foods.

Supplement savvy

It's so easy to get plenty of vitamin C from foods that extra supplements are not necessary, especially if you are already taking a multivitamin and mineral supplement.

Ascorbic acid is the most used and least expensive form of vitamin C in supplements. It is also the form most likely to cause stomach upset and erosion of tooth enamel. Calcium ascorbate and sodium ascorbate are available forms of vitamin C that are less likely to cause side effects.

Vitamin D

A stroll in the park, tending your garden or watching the children splash in the pool are some of the more pleasant ways to obtain vitamin D. Since you make your own vitamin D when you're in the sun, it's sometimes called the sunshine vitamin. There is concern that as more and more people use sunscreen to help prevent skin cancer, the rates for vitamin D deficiency may increase. Experts suggest that for most people it's okay to spend some time in the sun without sunscreen on your arms and legs (except from noon to 4 p.m.) to help increase vitamin D synthesis.

RECOMMENDED INTAKE

AI (Adequate Intake)

Vitamin D (mcg/d)

Life-Stage	Children	Men	Women	Pregnancy	Lactation
1-3 years	5				
4-8 years	5				
9-13 years	5			5	5
14-18 years		5	5	5	5
19-30 years		5	5	5	5
31-50 years		5	5	5	5
51-70 years		10	10		
70+ years		15	15		

Source: The National Academy of Sciences

WHAT IS IT?

Vitamin D really isn't a vitamin at all; it's a steroid hormone. It was originally misclassified as a fat-soluble vitamin, and to confuse matters even more, it's actually two separate calciferol (calcium-related) compounds: cholecalciferol and ergocalciferol. Exposing your skin to a sufficient amount of sunlight or artificial ultraviolet radiation can make each form of calciferol. Vitamin D's most important role is to regulate calcium levels in your body.

WHY YOU NEED IT

Bones & Teeth

Vitamin D is essential for helping calcium get into your bones. Without proper levels of vitamin D, you can't absorb enough calcium no matter how much you take in. Too little vitamin D can speed up the development of the crippling bone disease, osteoporosis. Occasionally, a vitamin D deficiency may cause slow, progressive hearing loss. If the bones in the inner ear become too weak or porous, they will not properly transmit sound waves. Sometimes, this special type of hearing loss can be improved with an adequate intake of vitamin D.

Heart & Circulatory System

Perhaps the most important muscle that needs calcium to work effectively is your heart. Vitamin D plays a critical role in regulating how much calcium stays in your blood.

Nervous System

Calcium is important for the transmission of nerve impulses and is required for muscle contraction.

MORE OR LESS?

Increased or decreased nutrient needs should always be discussed with your healthcare professional.

You may need higher than recommended levels of vitamin D if you have:

* *Darkly pigmented skin*
* *Diabetes*
* *Cystic fibrosis*
* *Gout*
* *Intestinal disease with diarrhea*
* *Kidney disease*
* *Liver disease*
* *Overactive thyroid function*
* *Disease of the pancreas*

You may also need higher than recommended levels of vitamin D if you:

* *Have been exposed to high levels of toxic chemicals at work*
* *Avoid the sun or are homebound*
* *Always use sunscreen*
* *Live in a community with high levels of air pollution*

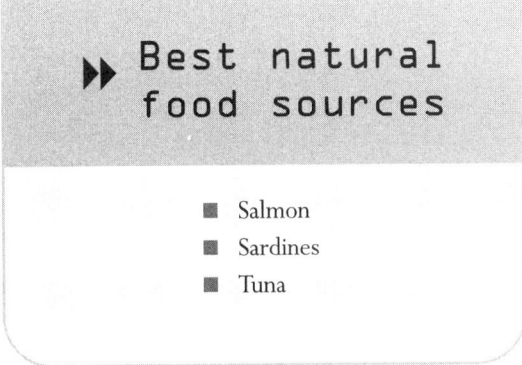

▶▶ Best natural food sources

- Salmon
- Sardines
- Tuna

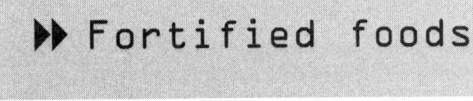

▶▶ Fortified foods

- Milk
- Margarine
- Some breakfast cereals

(Continued...)

41

IF YOU GET TOO LITTLE

Diarrhea, insomnia, nervousness and muscle twitching are some of the early signs of vitamin D deficiency. Bone weakening in children can lead to bone-deforming rickets, because newly formed bone lacks sufficient calcium. During pregnancy, too little vitamin D can cause osteomalacia, or adult rickets, in the pregnant woman.

IF YOU TAKE TOO MUCH

Excess vitamin D can cause constipation, headaches, nausea, high blood pressure, seizures, growth retardation and calcium deposits in the heart, blood vessels or kidneys. Minimum toxic dose is 1,000 IU or 25 mcg.

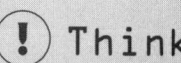 Think twice!

Never take more than 600 IU of vitamin D in supplemental form without a prescription from your healthcare provider.

Regular use of antacids containing magnesium taken with vitamin D supplements may result in high blood levels of magnesium, especially in people with kidney disease.

Taking thiazide diuretics (water pills) and vitamin D supplements may cause high blood levels of calcium and increase the chance of negative side effects.

 Did you know?

If you live in the southern half of the United States, chances are good that with regular outdoor time you can make and store plenty of vitamin D. If you live in the North, you should rely more on food sources of vitamin D.

Individuals with dark skin pigmentation have higher melanin content and require longer sun exposure to make vitamin D than people with light skin tones.

📄 Startling statistics

If you're over age 70, your ability to make vitamin D from sun exposure is reduced by half.

KITCHEN CONNECTIONS

✔ *Always choose dairy products fortified with vitamin D; check the nutrition facts panel.*
✔ *Add bran flakes (or other cereals fortified with vitamin D) into your favorite muffin mix or recipe.*

NUTRIENT THIEVES

▶ Mineral oil and laxative use can rob your body of fat-soluble vitamins, including vitamin D.
▶ Using sunscreen is very important to prevent your risk of skin cancer, but it can also block the sun's ability to produce vitamin D.

NORTH AFRICAN TUNA KABOBS

Fresh tuna is an outstanding source of vitamin D, and is absolutely delicious prepared this way. Serve these kabobs over couscous or rice and accompany with a selection of grilled vegetables.

½ cup chopped fresh cilantro
½ cup chopped fresh Italian parsley
4 garlic cloves, minced
½ cup extra-virgin olive oil
⅓ cup fresh lemon juice
2 teaspoons ground cumin
1½ teaspoons paprika
¾ teaspoon salt
½ teaspoon freshly ground pepper
1¾-lb. tuna steak (1¼ inches thick),
    cut into 1¼-inch chunks
2 lemons, each cut into 6 wedges

❶ In small bowl, whisk together cilantro, parsley, garlic, olive oil, lemon juice, cumin, paprika, salt and pepper. Reserve ½ cup of this mixture to serve as sauce. Place tuna in a shallow glass dish. Pour remaining marinade over tuna; turn to coat. Refrigerate, covered, at least 20 minutes or up to 1 hour, turning occasionally. Cover and keep reserved sauce at room temperature.

❷ Heat grill. Thread 1 piece of tuna, 1 lemon wedge, 2 pieces of tuna, another lemon wedge and final piece of tuna onto 10- or 12-inch skewer. Repeat with remaining tuna and lemon wedges to make a total of 6 kabobs.

❸ Lightly oil grill rack. Place kabobs on gas grill over high heat or on charcoal grill 4 to 6 inches from hot coals. Cover grill and cook, turning occasionally, 7 to 9 minutes or until tuna is browned and just begins to flake. Serve with reserved sauce.

6 servings.
Preparation time: 30 minutes.
Ready to serve: 1 hour.
Per serving: 300 calories, 20.5 g total fat (4 g saturated fat), 80 mg cholesterol, 295 mg sodium, 1 g fiber.

Vitamin E

If all the hype about vitamin E were true, you could live well past age 100 and have the sex drive and youthful appearance of a teenager. Vitamin E is no magical fountain of youth, but it does provide significant health benefits.

WHAT IS IT?

Vitamin E is really a group of fat-soluble compounds that are stored in fatty tissue throughout your body and in the liver. Its main function is the prevention of tissue breakdown. Unfortunately, vitamin E is one

RECOMMENDED INTAKE

RDA (Recommended Dietary Allowance)
Vitamin E (IU/d)

Life-Stage	Children	Men	Women	Pregnancy	Lactation
1-3 years	6				
4-8 years	7				
9-13 years	11			15	19
14-18 years		15	15	15	19
19-30 years		15	15	15	19
31-50 years		15	15	15	19
51-70 years		15	15		
70+ years		15	15		

Source: The National Academy of Sciences

For optimum health aim for 50 to 400 IU per day from foods or the natural form of the vitamin supplement.

nutrient that is difficult to obtain in optimal amounts from moderate-calorie foods.

WHY YOU NEED IT

Antioxidant Actions

Working as an antioxidant, vitamin E protects various tissues from destruction by free radicals (see pages 15–16 for more information). Vitamin E has been shown to help prevent age-related damage and deterioration to skin, blood vessels and the eyes.

Immune System

Vitamin E helps protect the thymus gland and circulating white blood cells from damage. It also helps protect immune function during chronic viral illness.

MORE OR LESS?

Increased or decreased nutrient needs should always be discussed with your healthcare professional.

You may need higher than recommended amounts of vitamin E if you:

* *Are age 50+*
* *Smoke*
* *Abuse alcohol*
* *Have been exposed to high levels of pollution*

▶▶ Fortified foods

- Some ready-to-eat cereals
- Some fruit juice drinks

IF YOU GET TOO LITTLE

It's rare to have a full-blown vitamin E deficiency. Symptoms may include fatigue, joint pain and muscular pain. In rare cases, low vitamin E levels have been linked to neurological damage and shortened life of red blood cells.

IF YOU TAKE TOO MUCH

Too much vitamin E can cause breast tenderness, depression, diarrhea, double vision, fatigue, intestinal cramping, gas, mood swings and weak muscles. High doses can also interfere with the effectiveness of anticoagulant (blood thinning) medicines prescribed to prevent blood clotting. Continued high intakes deplete vitamin A stores. The minimum toxic dose of vitamin E is 800 IU.

▶▶ Best natural food sources

- Almonds
- Hazelnuts
- Peanut butter
- Shrimp
- Sunflower seeds
- Wheat germ

(!) Think twice!

Antacids decrease vitamin E absorption. If you habitually take antacids, you will need supplemental vitamin E.

Use of mineral oil or laxatives will deplete fat-soluble vitamins, including vitamin E.

(Continued...)

Did you know?

In looking for better antioxidants, an international team of scientists stumbled onto a new form of vitamin E. Because oxidants can damage cells, many species load up their eggs with antioxidants, especially vitamins C and E. Researchers found that 20 percent of the vitamin E, or alpha-tocopherol, had an unexpected double bond at the end of its side chain where most alpha-tocopherol has a single bond. Newer studies have found the same structure in fish and plankton. The best news is that this different form of vitamin E seems to outperform the alpha-tocopherol structure.

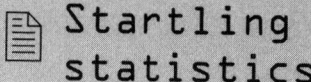 **Startling statistics**

It takes almost a pound of vegetables such as spinach, sweet potatoes or peas to provide just 20 to 30 IU of vitamin E. Oils, nuts and seeds are more concentrated sources of vitamin E, so choose them in moderation to avoid eating too many calories or grams of fat.

KITCHEN CONNECTIONS

✔ Dip bread lightly in olive oil instead of spreading it with butter.

✔ Toss some walnuts into your morning oatmeal or afternoon salad.

✔ Choose cold-pressed oils; they have higher levels of vitamin E.

NUTRIENT THIEVES

▶ Deep fat frying and reuse of cooking oils (frequently done in fast food and other restaurants) quickly depletes vitamin E levels. Most refined and processed grains have little of their original vitamin E content.

Supplement savvy

Vitamin E is the only nutrient where the "natural" form is preferable over synthetic versions. Ignore the product label and read the ingredient list. Look for d-alpha-tocopherol. If you see dl-alpha-tocopherol, it's the synthetic version. The extra "l" makes all the difference.

SHRIMP RISOTTO WITH LEMON & GARLIC

Parsley, lemon peel and garlic give this simple dish a special flourish, and shrimp offers plenty of vitamin E.

⅓ cup chopped fresh Italian parsley
1 teaspoon freshly grated lemon peel
2 medium garlic cloves, minced
2 (14.5-oz.) cans reduced-sodium chicken broth
½ cup water
4 teaspoons olive oil
12 oz. shelled, deveined uncooked medium shrimp,
    each cut into 2 or 3 pieces
2 medium shallots, finely chopped
Dash of crushed red pepper
1 cup Arborio rice
½ cup dry white wine
2 teaspoons fresh lemon juice
¼ teaspoon freshly ground pepper

1. In small bowl, combine parsley, lemon peel and garlic; toss with fork to mix.
2. In large saucepan, combine chicken broth and water; bring to a simmer over medium heat. Reduce heat to low; keep broth at low simmer.
3. In Dutch oven, heat 2 teaspoons oil over medium heat until hot. Add shrimp; cook about 2 minutes or until shrimp turn pink and opaque in center, stirring occasionally. Transfer to plate.
4. Add remaining 2 teaspoons oil to Dutch oven. Add shallots and red pepper; cook 30 seconds to 1 minute or until shallots are tender, stirring constantly. Add rice; cook 30 seconds, stirring constantly. Add wine; cook about 30 seconds or until almost evaporated, stirring constantly. Add 1 cup of the hot broth; cook 1 to 2 minutes or until most of the liquid has been absorbed, stirring constantly. Continue to simmer 18 to 20 minutes, stirring frequently, adding broth about ½ cup at a time and waiting until most of it has been absorbed before adding more, until rice is just tender and risotto has a creamy consistency.
5. Add shrimp; cook about 1 minute or until heated through. Remove risotto from heat. Stir in parsley mixture, lemon juice and pepper.

4 (1¼-cup) servings.
Preparation time: 15 minutes.
Ready to serve: 40 minutes.
Per serving: 335 calories, 7 g total fat (1.5 g saturated fat), 120 mg cholesterol, 570 mg sodium, 1 g fiber.

Vitamin K

orldwide, only a handful of researchers study vitamin K, which is known for its critical role in blood clotting. But with the aging of the American population, this vitamin may rate a bigger following as its importance to the integrity of bones becomes increasingly clear.

WHAT IS IT?

Vitamin K is a fat-soluble vitamin. The vitamin K present in plant foods is called phylloquinone; the form of the vitamin present in animal foods is called menaquinone. Both of these vitamins are absorbed

RECOMMENDED INTAKE

AI (Adequate Intake)

Vitamin K (mcg/d)

Life-Stage	Children	Men	Women	Pregnancy	Lactation
1-3 years	30				
4-8 years	55				
9-13 years	60			75	75
14-18 years		75	75	75	75
19-30 years		120	90	90	90
31-50 years		120	90	90	90
51-70 years		120	90		
70+ years		120	90		

Source: The National Academy of Sciences

The suggested intake for optimal health is 65 to 200 mcg per day.

and converted to an active form called dihydrovitamin K. Bacteria living in the intestines supply a portion of your vitamin K needs. Most Americans consume about three to five times more than the RDA of vitamin K and deficiencies are quite rare.

WHY YOU NEED IT

Bones & Teeth

Vitamin K helps maintain healthy bone tissue and activates at least three proteins involved in bone health. It is also a critical part of the healing process after bone fractures.

Circulatory System

The most well known function of vitamin K is the key role it plays in helping control blood clotting by the production of prothrombin.

MORE OR LESS?

You might need more vitamin K if you:
* *Are on long-term antibiotic therapy*
* *Have a fat metabolism disorder*
* *Take oral contraceptives*
* *Regularly exercise heavily; are a professional or a very active athlete in training*
* *Are age 70 or older*

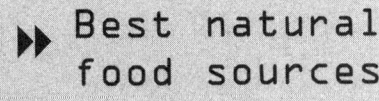

Best natural food sources

- Asparagus
- Broccoli
- Brussels sprouts
- Cabbage
- Collard greens
- Endive
- Green apples
- Kale
- Red leaf lettuce
- Swiss chard
- Watercress

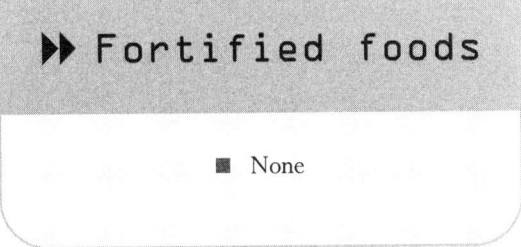

Fortified foods

- None

IF YOU GET TOO LITTLE

Vitamin K deficiency is very rare. It occurs when there is an inability to absorb the vitamin from the intestinal tract. Vitamin K deficiency can also occur after prolonged treatment with oral antibiotics.

IF YOU TAKE TOO MUCH

There are no reported cases of healthy individuals having side effects with large amounts of vitamin K. However, excess vitamin K may cause impaired liver function in those with advanced liver disease.

(Continued...)

Think twice!

You don't have to give up nutrient-rich foods like leafy green vegetables if you take Coumadin medication to prevent blood clots. You don't need a diet low in vitamin K; you need a diet with a consistent daily intake of vitamin K. Your doctor can adjust your medications to accommodate your intake of this healthy nutrient.

KITCHEN CONNECTIONS

✔ *Think green!*
✔ *Add broccoli or asparagus to pasta.*
✔ *Serve sliced green apples with cheese.*
✔ *Add colorful and flavorful endive to salad.*

NUTRIENT THIEVES

▸ Little vitamin K is lost from foods during ordinary cooking.

▸ Use of mineral oil or laxatives will deplete fat-soluble vitamins, including vitamin E.

 Did you know?

If you've ever had a baby, you might remember that almost all newborns are given an injection of vitamin K shortly before they leave the hospital. That's because newborns are born with a sterile intestinal tract and have not yet developed normal, healthy bacteria to produce vitamin K.

Supplement savvy

Vitamin K supplements are not recommended for most people.

If you want more vitamin K in your diet, try alfalfa tablets. Remember, however, that to be absorbed, vitamin K must be consumed with fat.

 Startling statistics

A single large salad of dark leafy greens each day can provide all the extra vitamin K you need.

SESAME ASPARAGUS

So many vegetables offer vitamin K ... why not try some asparagus prepared this wonderful, Asian way.

1 tablespoon oyster sauce
1 tablespoon soy sauce
1 tablespoon dry sherry or white wine
1 teaspoon cornstarch
1½ teaspoons dark sesame oil
2 tablespoons sesame seeds
1 tablespoon vegetable oil
1½ teaspoons minced fresh ginger
1 teaspoon minced garlic
1 lb. asparagus, trimmed, cut
    diagonally into 1½-inch pieces
1 large carrot, cut diagonally into thin pieces
½ cup chicken broth or water
1 bunch green onions, cut
    diagonally into 1-inch pieces

❶ In small bowl, combine oyster sauce, soy sauce and sherry. Add cornstarch; stir to dissolve. Stir in sesame oil. Set aside.

❷ Place sesame seeds in unheated wok. Brown over medium heat until seeds turn golden, about 2 to 3 minutes. Remove seeds; set aside. Increase heat to high. Add oil; swirl to coat wok. Add ginger, garlic, asparagus and carrot. Stir-fry 2 minutes. Add broth; cover and cook an additional 2 minutes or until asparagus and carrot are almost crisp-tender. Uncover. Add green onions. Stir-fry an additional minute. Add oyster sauce mixture; stir until thickened. Toss with sesame seeds.

4 servings.
Preparation time: 30 minutes.
Ready to serve: 30 minutes.
Per serving: 125 calories, 8 g total fat (1 g saturated fat), 0 mg cholesterol, 575 mg sodium, 3 g fiber.

Thiamin
or Vitamin B1

Thiamin was the first B vitamin discovered, and hence was named Vitamin B1. It was named to reflect the Greek word for sulfur, *thio*, since this complicated molecule has an atom of sulfur attached.

RECOMMENDED INTAKE
RDA (Recommended Dietary Allowance)
Thiamin (mg/d)

Life-Stage	Children	Men	Women	Pregnancy	Lactation
1-3 years	0.5				
4-8 years	0.6				
9-13 years	0.9			1.4	1.4
14-18 years		1.0	1.0	1.4	1.4
19-30 years		1.1	1.1	1.4	1.4
31-50 years		1.1	1.1	1.4	1.4
51-70 years		1.1	1.1		
70+ years		1.1	1.1		

Source: The National Academy of Sciences

WHAT IS IT?

Thiamin, or vitamin B1, is water-soluble and functions as part of an enzyme (thiamin pyrophosphate) essential for energy production, carbohydrate metabolism and nerve function. Thiamin is found in both plant and animal foods.

WHY YOU NEED IT

Metabolism
Thiamin helps stabilize the appetite by improving digestion, particularly that of sugars, starches and alcohol. Some thiamin is stored in the heart, liver and kidneys, but these stores do not last long and a continuous intake is necessary to prevent deficiency.

Nervous System & Brain
Thiamin helps maintain a healthy nervous system and positive mental attitude. Thiamin's coenzyme form is also utilized in the synthesis of acetylcholine. A lack of acetlycholine causes inflammation of the nerves, and memory loss. Thiamin is also involved with improving learning capacity and is necessary for general growth and development in children.

MORE OR LESS?

Increased or decreased nutrient needs should always be discussed with your healthcare professional.

You might need more thiamin if you are:

* *Age 70 or older*
* *A person with Alzheimer's*
* *An alcohol abuser*
* *Epileptic*
* *A routine heavy exerciser*

▶▶ Best natural food sources

- Ham
- Pompano fish
- Pork
- Sunflower seeds

▶▶ Fortified foods

- Bread
- Hot cereals
- Pasta
- Ready-to-eat cold cereals
- Rice

IF YOU GET TOO LITTLE

Symptoms of mild thiamin deficiency include fatigue, depression, constipation and tingling or numbness of the legs. Older people in hospitals and nursing homes seem to be at highest risk for deficiency. Severe deficiency of thiamin results in wet or dry beriberi. Wet beriberi is characterized by the accumulation of fluids in the tissues, especially in the ankles, legs and feet. This edema affects cardiovascular function, and can be fatal. There is no fluid accumulation in dry beriberi, but there is severe muscle atrophy, significant weight loss and paralysis of the legs. Both types of beriberi may include symptoms of mental confusion and difficulty walking.

(Continued...)

53

IF YOU TAKE TOO MUCH

It's rare to overdose on thiamin. Some symptoms you are taking too much include dark urine, nausea or vomiting. Minimum toxic dose is 1 gram.

Think twice!

Raw freshwater fish and shellfish contain an enzyme that breaks down thiamin. This can happen during food storage and preparation or as food passes through the stomach. Thus, large intakes of raw fish and shellfish can increase the risk of thiamin deficiency.

Did you know?

Thiamin functions as a coenzyme in the complex process of converting glucose (blood sugar) into energy and is vital in certain metabolic reactions. For this reason, thiamin is needed during exercise and times of high-energy expenditure.

Startling statistics

Beriberi is still common in many parts of Asia, where white rice is a major staple.

KITCHEN CONNECTIONS

✔ *Use enriched or whole-grain pasta or rice and do not wash before cooking or rinse after cooking.*
✔ *Roast meat at a moderate temperature and cook only until it is done—overcooking at a high temperature destroys thiamin.*
✔ *Top low-fat yogurt with crunchy wheat germ.*
✔ *Sprinkle fresh soybeans or peas into pasta salads.*
✔ *Substitute polenta instead of potatoes for a side dish.*

NUTRIENT THIEVES

▶ Alcohol interferes with the absorption of all nutrients, but especially thiamin.
▶ A diet containing excessive amounts of sugar may cause marginal thiamin deficiency.
▶ Thiamin is vulnerable to heat during cooking.
▶ Drinking large quantities of tea and coffee may reduce thiamin absorption.

Supplement savvy

It is generally recommended to take B vitamins as a complete B complex, because large doses of any single B vitamin may, over time, cause a B complex imbalance. All good multivitamins contain all the extra B nutrients most people need.

PORK CHOPS WITH DRIED-APPLE STUFFING

Pork is an excellent source of thiamin, and this healthy recipe cooks it up in a taste-filled, down-home way. Choose chops ¾ to 1 inch thick.

½ cup dried apples, cut into ½-inch pieces
½ cup apple cider or apple juice
3 tablespoons vegetable oil
3 large shallots, chopped
¼ cup chopped celery
1 cup fresh brown bread crumbs
¾ teaspoon dried sage
4 (8-oz.) center-cut pork chops
⅛ teaspoon each salt, freshly ground pepper
¼ cup water

❶ Place apples in small bowl; pour cider over apples. Microwave on High power 1½ minutes; drain and set aside, reserving liquid.

❷ In medium skillet, heat 2 tablespoons oil over medium-high heat until hot. Sauté shallots and celery until shallots begin to brown. Remove from heat. Add bread crumbs, sage, well-drained dried apples and just enough apple liquid to moisten; mix well.

❸ Heat broiler. Cut pocket in each pork chop*. Stuff mixture into pockets. Brush with remaining oil; sprinkle with salt and pepper. Arrange in 13x9-inch pan; place under broiler 1 to 2 minutes or until brown.

❹ Heat oven to 350°F. Secure stuffed pockets with toothpicks. Pour water into pan; cover tightly with aluminum foil. Bake 30 minutes. Uncover and bake an additional 20 minutes or until internal temperature reaches at least 160°F.

TIP *Make a pocket by using a sharp knife to cut toward the bone.

4 servings.
Preparation time: 15 minutes.
Ready to serve: 1 hour, 15 minutes.
Per serving: 550 calories, 30 g fat (8.5 g saturated fat), 100 mg cholesterol, 380 mg sodium, 2.5 g fiber.

Riboflavin or Vitamin B2

The luminous yellow-green color patterns that shimmer in milk, whey, liver and eggs are what first attracted scientists to investigate what was later called riboflavin. View your eggs or milk at just the right angle and you too can see the glorious rainbow of colors.

RECOMMENDED INTAKE

AI (Adequate Intake)

Riboflavin (mg/d)

Life-Stage	Children	Men	Women	Pregnancy	Lactation
1-3 years	0.5				
4-8 years	0.6				
9-13 years	0.9			1.4	1.6
14-18 years		1.3	1.0	1.4	1.6
19-30 years		1.3	1.1	1.4	1.6
31-50 years		1.3	1.1	1.4	1.6
51-70 years		1.3	1.1		
70+ years		1.3	1.1		

Source: The National Academy of Sciences

What Is It?

Riboflavin is a coenzyme (that is, the non-protein, active part of an enzyme). Unlike many other nutrients, riboflavin is easily absorbed from foods. Riboflavin is an exception to the water-soluble vitamin rule, because you do store small amounts of it in your kidneys and liver.

Why You Need It

Energy Production
Riboflavin provides energy at the most basic level—your cells. Every cell needs riboflavin to release energy from protein, carbohydrates and fat.

Hormones
Riboflavin is important in the production of thyroid hormones and in adrenal gland function.

Immune System
Riboflavin aids in the production of infection-fighting immune cells.

Nervous System
Nerve development and brain neurotransmitters require the presence of riboflavin.

More or Less?

Increased or decreased nutrient needs should always be discussed with your healthcare professional.
You may need higher than recommended amounts of riboflavin if you are:
* *Age 70 or older*
* *An alcohol abuser*
* *On long-term antibiotic therapy*
* *Taking oral contraceptives*
* *Having renal dialysis*
* *Pregnant with two or more fetuses*

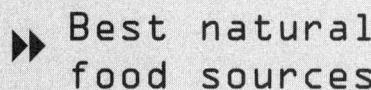

▶▶ Best natural food sources

- ■ Buttermilk
- ■ Milk
- ■ Yogurt

▶▶ Fortified foods

- ■ Bread
- ■ Pasta
- ■ Rice
- ■ Some ready-to-eat cold cereals

If You Get Too Little

If you eat lots of overly refined foods you may not get enough riboflavin. The most common symptoms of riboflavin deficiency include inflammation of the mouth and tongue. Small cracks and fissures at the corners of your mouth may also be a telltale sign of deficiency. Increased sensitivity to light and a purplish tongue are also symptoms of a diet low in riboflavin.

If You Take Too Much

Bright yellow urine is the most common side effect of taking too much riboflavin. Nausea and vomiting may also result. Minimum toxic dose is not known.

(Continued...)

! Think twice!

If you don't drink milk, you may be at risk for a marginal riboflavin deficiency. If you are allergic to milk, eat plenty of dark, leafy green vegetables. If you are lactose intolerant, try to consume small amounts of dairy products throughout the day or consider taking a chewable lactase supplement (like Lactaid or Dairy Ease) just before you eat dairy foods.

? Did you know?

Milk is no longer widely available in clear glass bottles because milk can lose up to 75 percent of its riboflavin when exposed to light for just a few hours. Milk packed in cardboard or opaque plastic containers is shielded from light at the grocery store and in your refrigerator. Some milk companies have changed to thicker, denser plastic jugs to add even more protection.

📄 Startling statistics

Riboflavin is activated in your liver. Major tranquilizers and long-term use of barbiturates may interfere with the process.

KITCHEN CONNECTIONS

✔ Use plain yogurt instead of mayonnaise in a sauce or dip recipe.
✔ Add dark turkey meat to a salad or sandwich.
✔ Make a fruit smoothie with skim milk.

NUTRIENT THIEVES

▶ Light and heat are the most harmful agents to riboflavin. Food can lose up to 75 percent of its riboflavin when cooked.

Supplement savvy

It is generally recommended that you take B vitamins as a complete B complex, because large doses of any single B vitamin may, over time, cause a B complex imbalance. All good multivitamins contain all the riboflavin most people need.

CHICKEN & VEGETABLES WITH PASTA

Here's a versatile recipe with many vitamin-filled ingredients. Branch out and select different pasta varieties, and use any vegetables that are in season.

8 oz. multicolored rotelle or penne rigate pasta
2 tablespoons olive oil
1 lb. boneless skinless chicken breast halves,
   rinsed and cut into 1-inch pieces
1 garlic clove, minced
5 cups seasonal vegetables*
4 green onions, chopped
¼ can sun-dried tomatoes, packed in oil, drained
6 plum tomatoes, diced (½ inch thick)
1 teaspoon dried basil
½ teaspoon pepper
2 teaspoons freshly grated lemon peel
1 tablespoon fresh lemon juice
Freshly grated Parmesan cheese
Toasted pine nuts

❶ Cook pasta according to package directions. Drain.

❷ Meanwhile, in heavy skillet, heat 1 tablespoon oil over medium-high heat until hot. Add chicken; cook, about 4 minutes or until chicken is no longer pink in center. Set aside.

❸ Add remaining 1 tablespoon oil, garlic, vegetables and onions to skillet; toss over high heat 4 to 6 minutes or until vegetables are tender. Reduce heat to low. Stir in chicken, tomatoes, basil and pepper; cook about 1 minute or until chicken is warm. Remove from heat; add lemon peel and juice.

❹ Toss pasta with chicken and vegetables. Serve with Parmesan cheese and toasted pine nuts.

TIP *Seasonal vegetables may include: zucchini, broccoli florets, fresh asparagus and carrots julienne.

4 servings.
Preparation time: 10 minutes.
Ready to serve: 25 minutes.
Per serving: 555 calories, 19 g total fat (4 g saturated fat), 65 mg cholesterol, 450 mg sodium, 7.5 g fiber.

Niacin or Vitamin B3

The deficiency disease pellagra was rampant in the United States during the Great Depression when protein-rich foods such as meat, poultry, fish and eggs were scarce. Today, the increased availability of protein-rich foods has all but eliminated pellagra.

RECOMMENDED INTAKE

RDA (Recommended Dietary Allowance)

Niacin (mg/d)

Life-Stage	Children	Men	Women	Pregnancy	Lactation
1-3 years	6				
4-8 years	8				
9-13 years	12			18	17
14-18 years		16	14	18	17
19-30 years		16	14	18	17
31-50 years		16	14	18	17
51-70 years		16	14		
70+ years		16	14		

Source: The National Academy of Sciences

WHAT IS IT?

Niacin is actually the generic name for two similar substances—nicotinic acid and nicotinamide—neither of which are related to the nicotine in cigarettes. Niacin is involved in more than 200 enzyme reactions in your body. Water-soluble niacin is found in foods, but can also be converted from the amino acid tryptophan if you have plenty of iron, riboflavin and vitamin B6 available.

WHY YOU NEED IT

Circulation
Niacin helps relax and loosen blood vessels.

Hormones
Niacin is required in the formation of a variety of hormones including sex hormones, cortisone, thyroxin and insulin. An abundance of niacin also helps your body quickly notice and respond to insulin released after eating.

Nervous System
Niacin plays an essential role in the normal functioning of your brain and nervous system.

MORE OR LESS?

Increased or decreased nutrient needs should always be discussed with your healthcare professional.

You may need higher than recommended amounts of niacin if you have:
* *Hartnup's disease—a genetic disorder that affects tryptophan absorption*
* *A vegetarian diet that includes no animal products or by-products*

▶▶ Best natural food sources

- Chicken
- Lamb
- Pork
- Veal
- Mackerel
- Mullet
- Salmon
- Swordfish

▶▶ Fortified foods

- Breads
- Cereals
- Pasta

IF YOU GET TOO LITTLE

Weakness, loss of appetite, irritability and confusion are early signs of low levels of niacin. In some people, a red rash that looks like sunburn may appear and the tongue may turn bright red. The three D's identify the deficiency disease called pellagra: dementia (loss or decrease in mental function), diarrhea and dermatitis.

(Continued...)

IF YOU TAKE TOO MUCH

A common side effect of using niacin therapy to lower blood cholesterol is skin flushing. Time-released niacin supplements were developed to help reduce this effect, but these slow-absorbing formulas have been found to be more toxic to the liver. Amounts as low as 50 mg per day of niacin can produce flushing if taken on an empty stomach. Doses of 500 mg or more may cause high blood sugar, itching, irregular heart rhythm, nausea or ulcers. Blurred vision, eye and eyelid swelling and loss of eyebrows and eyelashes are also common side effects of too much niacin.

(!) Think twice!

If you have liver disease, gout, high blood pressure, peptic ulcers or a high intake of alcohol, niacin supplements are not recommended.

Niacin therapy should only be used in people with significantly high blood cholesterol levels. Don't take niacin in large amounts without medical guidance.

(?) Did you know?

Claims that niacin is effective for treatment of acne, alcoholism, unwanted effects of drug abuse, leprosy, motion sickness, muscle problems, poor circulation and mental problems, and for prevention of heart attacks, have not been proven. Many of these treatments involve large and expensive amounts of vitamins.

When corn became a staple food in the early 1700s in Europe, pellagra reached epidemic proportions. Reliance on corn foods in the southeastern United States in the early 1900s sparked our own pellagra epidemic. A protein molecule bound to the niacin in corn prevents niacin absorption, which leads to pellagra. In 1941, the federal grain enrichment program was developed as a response to the devastation caused by pellagra. Today, many corn-based products like tortillas are soaked in limewater, which releases the niacin and makes it useable.

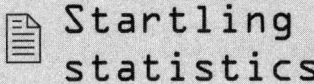

KITCHEN CONNECTIONS

- ✔ *Enjoy a pecan- or almond-encrusted salmon or swordfish fillet.*
- ✔ *Add some flaked tuna to a leafy green salad.*
- ✔ *Choose whole grain breads and cereals for extra niacin.*

Pyridoxine or Vitamin B6

Pyridoxine's claim to fame came in the early 1980s when it was proclaimed the pre-menstrual syndrome (PMS) vitamin. It didn't take long—just until 1983—to see the first descriptions of toxicity described in the *New England Journal of Medicine*. Even today, many physicians and clinics that

RECOMMENDED INTAKE
RDA (Recommended Dietary Allowance)
Vitamin B6 (mg/d)

Life-Stage	Children	Men	Women	Pregnancy	Lactation
1-3 years	0.5				
4-8 years	0.6				
9-13 years	1.0			1.4	1.6
14-18 years		1.3	1.2	1.4	1.6
19-30 years		1.3	1.3	1.4	1.6
31-50 years		1.3	1.3	1.4	1.6
51-70 years		1.7	1.5		
70+ years		1.7	1.5		

Source: The National Academy of Sciences

specialize in treating PMS routinely prescribe potentially toxic levels of B6, up to 2,000 mg per day.

WHAT IS IT?

Vitamin B6 is a water-soluble vitamin that has three forms: pyridoxine, pyridoxal and pyridoxamine. It performs a wide variety of functions and is essential for overall good health. More than 60 different enzymes depend on B6 for activation.

WHY YOU NEED IT

Circulatory System
Vitamin B6 helps your body maintain normal homocysteine levels that can lower your risk for heart disease.

Metabolism
The most important function of vitamin B6 is protein metabolism. It helps cells figure out which amino acids to break down for energy and which to convert into other amino acids. This nutrient also helps maintain the chemical balance of body fluids and regulates water excretion.

Nervous System
Vitamin B6 is crucial in making key nervous system regulators or neurotransmitters. The link between B6 and neurotransmitters is what started the PMS research.

MORE OR LESS?

Increased or decreased nutrient needs should always be discussed with your healthcare professional.

You may need higher than recommended amounts of vitamin B6 if you:

* Smoke
* Use oral contraceptives
* Are age 70 or older
* Have elevated homocysteine levels
* Abuse alcohol
* Abuse drugs

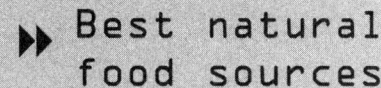

▶▶ Best natural food sources

- ■ Bananas
- ■ Chicken
- ■ Mangoes
- ■ Plantains
- ■ Wheat bran
- ■ Wheat germ

▶▶ Fortified foods

- ■ Oatmeal
- ■ Ready-to-eat cereals

IF YOU GET TOO LITTLE

Low levels of B6 have many of the common symptoms of a poor diet. These include weakness, poor appetite, dermatitis and increased susceptibility to infection.

IF YOU TAKE TOO MUCH

Taken over time, 200 mg or more of vitamin B6 may cause physiological dependence, which leads to undesirable higher needs. Other symptoms include night restlessness, sun sensitivity and an acne-like rash. Amounts of 500 mg or more may cause nerve disorders, pain, numbness, sun-induced skin rash, weakness or paralysis in your limbs. Too much vitamin B6 may also cause depression when large amounts are taken with oral contraceptives.

(Continued...)

(!) Think twice!

Large amounts of B6 can cause the anti-seizure drug Dilantin to break down too quickly. Check with your healthcare professional if you want to take B6 or a B vitamin complex supplement.

 ## (?) Did you know?

Most fruits and vegetables do not have much B6.

 ## Supplement savvy

Vitamin B6 is one water-soluble nutrient that requires extra caution when choosing supplements. Too much B6 can cause permanent neurological problems that may impair your ability to walk. Stick to the amount of B6 in a multivitamin supplement. As with all B complex vitamins, it's not smart to take individual pills—this family of nutrients works best as a group.

KITCHEN CONNECTIONS

✔ *Slice up some bananas or exotic plantains to top cereal or, even better, oatmeal.*
✔ *Make a Thai peanut sauce for stir-fry.*
✔ *Include wheat germ in breading for crispy oven-baked chicken.*
✔ *Add wheat bran to muffin, pancake and waffle batters.*

NUTRIENT THIEVES

▸ The higher your protein intake, the higher your need for vitamin B6.
▸ Freezing can destroy up to 70 percent of the B6 in foods.

CHICKEN MARINATED IN YOGURT WITH LEMON AND PEPPER

This grilled chicken is delicious as well as low in fat. And the long, slow marinating in garlicky yogurt tenderizes, moistens and adds flavor. Plus, chicken is a great source of vitamin B6. Serve with steamed rice and soft pita bread or flatbread.

2 large garlic cloves, minced
½ teaspoon salt
2 cups plain whole-milk yogurt
¼ cup lemon juice
Pulp of 1 large lemon
½ teaspoon freshly ground pepper
2 large bone-in chicken breasts

❶ In large shallow bowl, stir together garlic, salt, yogurt, lemon juice, lemon pulp and pepper. Remove skin and fat from chicken. Rinse chicken and pat dry. Bend breasts backward to break bones so pieces lie flat. Add chicken to yogurt mixture; turn to coat all sides.

❷ Cover bowl tightly; refrigerate at least overnight, turning once or twice.

❸ Remove chicken from marinade; discard. Place on gas grill over medium-high heat or on charcoal grill 4 to 6 inches from medium coals. Cook 12 to 16 minutes on each side or until no longer pink in center, turning once. Meat should be well browned but not burned.

6 servings.
Preparation time: 30 minutes.
Ready to serve: 12 hours.
Per serving: 140 calories, 3.5 g total fat (1.5 g saturated fat), 62 mg cholesterol, 110 mg sodium, 0 g fiber.

Folic Acid
or Vitamin B9

Smart Nutrition

olic acid has earned the honor of contributing the most striking public health improvement of any vitamin this decade. As more women learn of the link between folic acid and prevention of birth defects, the number of babies born with spina bifida has decreased. Evidence is mounting that optimal levels of folic acid may also help reduce heart disease by controlling the amount of

RECOMMENDED INTAKE

RDA (Recommended Dietary Allowance)

Folic Acid (mcg/d)

Life-Stage	Children	Men	Women	Pregnancy	Lactation
1-3 years	150				
4-8 years	200				
9-13 years	300			600	500
14-18 years		400	400	600	500
19-30 years		400	400	600	500
31-50 years		400	400	600	500
51-70 years		400	400		
70+ years		400	400		

Source: The National Academy of Sciences

homocysteine in the blood. High levels of this amino acid can damage artery walls and speed the buildup of plaque.

WHAT IS IT?

Folic acid is a water-soluble nutrient. Folate and folic acid are interchangeable terms. Folic acid is the synthetic form of folate, which is found naturally in foods. Popeye fans will be pleased to know that folic acid was first discovered in spinach.

WHY YOU NEED IT

Immune System
Folic acid is a vital component of white blood cell manufacture, which helps the functioning of your immune system.

Nervous System & Brain
Folic acid is involved in the production of neuro-transmitters such as serotonin and dopamine, which regulate brain functions including mood, sleep and appetite. Folic acid is essential for the development of the brain, spinal cord and skeleton in the fetus.

Metabolism
Folic acid is essential for protein metabolism. It converts the amino acid known as homocysteine to methionine. High levels of homocysteine have been linked to an increased risk of cardiovascular disease. Around 50 percent of body stores are in the liver. The amount stored may last for about four months before symptoms of deficiency develop.

MORE OR LESS?

Increased or decreased nutrient needs should always be discussed with your healthcare professional.
    You may need higher than recommended amounts of folic acid if you:
* *Are age 70 or older*
* *Take oral contraceptives*
* *Have high homocysteine levels*

▶▶ Best natural food sources

- Asparagus
- Black-eyed peas
- Kidney beans
- Lentils
- Oatmeal
- Orange juice
- Pinto beans
- Spinach (cooked)

▶▶ Fortified foods

- Bread
- Pasta
- Ready-to-eat cold or hot cereals
- Rice

IF YOU GET TOO LITTLE

When folic acid intake is inadequate, the levels in red blood cells fall, homocysteine concentration rises and finally, changes in the blood cell-producing bone marrow and other rapidly dividing cells occur. Ultimately, folic acid deficiency affects the growth and repair of all the cells and tissues of the body. Too little folic acid during early pregnancy is the leading cause of the birth defect spina bifida.

(Continued...)

IF YOU TAKE TOO MUCH

Fever, general weakness or discomfort, reddened skin, shortness of breath, skin rash or itching, tightness in chest, troubled breathing and wheezing are all signs that you're taking too much folic acid. Toxicity is considered rare. Symptoms are gastrointestinal disturbances, sleep problems and possible allergic skin reactions. Minimum toxic dose is 15 mg.

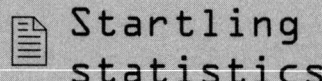

Startling statistics

You only absorb about half of the folic acid you eat, but folic acid used in fortified foods is absorbed at a much higher rate.

(!) Think twice!

Daily doses of more than 400 micrograms of folic acid can hide symptoms of pernicious anemia and counteract medications used to prevent epileptic seizures.

Large amounts of folic acid can mask anemia caused by vitamin B12 deficiency. Although this is rare, too little folic acid may lead to permanent nerve damage in some cases.

KITCHEN CONNECTIONS

✔ *Add beet juice to a marinade, dressing or sauce.*
✔ *Add okra or chickpeas to rice pilaf.*
✔ *Include great northern beans in soup or stew.*
✔ *Toss flavorful arugula into salads, cold pasta and wrap sandwiches.*

NUTRIENT THIEVES

▶ Folic acid is one of the most fragile B vitamins and can be completely destroyed in foods when exposed to air, light or heat for any extended period of time.

▶ Keeping foods uncovered at room temperature for long periods can also destroy folic acid.

(?) Did you know?

In 1998, the FDA required that bread, flour, cornmeal, rice, noodles, pasta and other grain products be fortified with folic acid. The goal was to make sure that most Americans got at least 400 micrograms a day from foods. According to a report in the *New England Journal of Medicine* one year later, the number of people with low folic acid levels in one study dropped by 92 percent.

Supplement savvy

Look for multivitamin/mineral supplements that provide exactly 400 micrograms of folic acid—no more, no less. As with all B complex vitamins, it's not smart to take individual pills since this family of nutrients works best as a group.

GREEK LENTIL SALAD

Small green lentils, loaded with folic acid, are preferred for salads because they retain their shape and have an appealing, chewy texture. Common brown lentils are a reasonable substitute. This salad makes a satisfying lunch or the perfect filling for a pita or other sandwich.

LEMON VINAIGRETTE
1 garlic clove, crushed
½ teaspoon salt
3 tablespoons fresh lemon juice
2 tablespoons extra-virgin olive oil
¼ teaspoon freshly ground pepper

SALAD
1 cup green or brown lentils, rinsed
½ teaspoon salt
1 cup trimmed chopped scallions
1 (12-oz.) jar roasted red bell peppers,
    rinsed, diced
½ cup (2 oz.) crumbled feta cheese
⅓ cup chopped fresh dill
6 cups torn arugula

1 In mortar and pestle or with side of chef's knife, mash garlic and ½ teaspoon salt into a paste; transfer to small bowl. Whisk in lemon juice, oil and pepper.

2 In large saucepan, cover lentils with water. Bring to a simmer over medium-high heat. Reduce heat to medium-low. Simmer, partially covered, 15 minutes. Add ½ teaspoon salt; cook an additional 5 to 10 minutes or just until lentils are tender but not broken down. Drain and cool slightly.

3 In large bowl, combine warm lentils and vinaigrette. Toss gently to mix. Add scallions, roasted peppers, feta and dill to lentil mixture; toss again. (Salad can be prepared up to 8 hours ahead. Cover and refrigerate. Bring to room temperature before serving.) To serve, mound lentil mixture on a bed of arugula.

8 (½-cup) servings.
Preparation time: 20 minutes.
Ready to serve: 45 minutes.
Per serving: 150 calories, 5.5 g total fat (1.5 g saturated fat), 5 mg cholesterol, 355 mg sodium, 6.5 g fiber.

Cobalamin
or Vitamin B12

Cobalamin can sometimes be considered a true miracle cure. Picture an elderly woman admitted to the hospital with symptoms of senility. She is frail, but was able to care for herself, carry on intelligent conversations and answer common questions. Gradually, her mental

RECOMMENDED INTAKE

RDA (Recommended Dietary Allowance)

Vitamin B12 (mcg/d)

Life-Stage	Children	Men	Women	Pregnancy	Lactation
1-3 years	0.9				
4-8 years	1.2				
9-13 years	1.8			2.6	2.8
14-18 years		2.4	2.4	2.6	2.8
19-30 years		2.4	2.4	2.6	2.8
31-50 years		2.4	2.4	2.6	2.8
51-70 years		2.4	2.4		
70+ years		2.4	2.4		

Source: The National Academy of Sciences

abilities faded to the point that Alzheimer's or senility was considered. After ruling out these and other serious problems, a simple injection of vitamin B12 led to sudden, dramatic improvements. She's up, walking the halls of her hospital wing, smiling and is "back to normal." That's quite an impact!

How does B12 effect this improvement? As humans age, our bodies naturally make less of the substance called "intrinsic factor," which helps us absorb vitamin B12. Injections or large doses of B12 help stimulate how much can be absorbed and can result in rapid neurological improvement.

WHAT IS IT?

Vitamin B12 was the last B complex vitamin to be discovered. It's a water-soluble nutrient that binds with a substance called intrinsic factor (a protein produced in your stomach lining) before being absorbed in your intestines. Low levels of stomach acid or too little intrinsic factor can lead to deficiencies of B12.

WHY YOU NEED IT

Circulatory System
Normal red blood cell production and function rely on vitamin B12.

Immune System
Too little vitamin B12 leads to a reduction in the number of white blood cells, which help fight infection.

Metabolism
You need vitamin B12 to help metabolize both fat and carbohydrates. B12 helps the formation of amino acid chains to make protein. Rapidly growing cells such as bone marrow and the outer layers of skin need B12 more than other cells.

Nervous System & Brain
The coating of nerve tissue, the myelin sheath, is made with help from vitamin B12. It is also essential in the formation of transmitters that send nerve impulses.

MORE OR LESS?

Increased or decreased nutrient needs should always be discussed with your healthcare professional.

You may need higher than recommended amounts of vitamin B12 if you are age 60 or older, if you maintain a strict vegetarian or macrobiotic diet or if you have:

* *Alcoholism*
* *Genetic disorders such as homocystinuria and/or methylmalonic aciduria*
* *Infections (continuing or chronic)*
* *Intestinal disease*
* *Kidney disease*
* *Liver disease*
* *Pancreatic disease*
* *Stomach disease*
* *Thyroid disease*

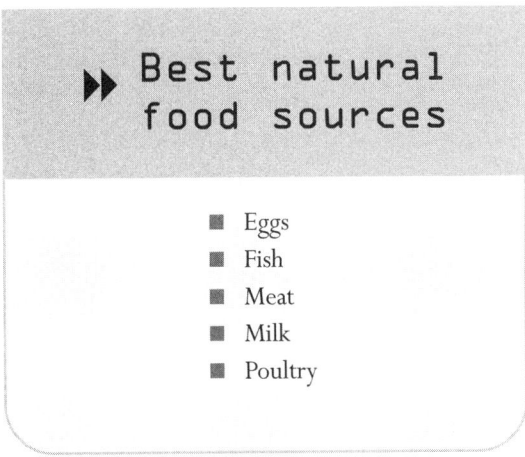

▶▶ Best natural food sources

- Eggs
- Fish
- Meat
- Milk
- Poultry

(Continued...)

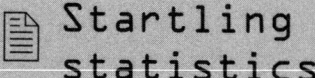

▶▶ Fortified foods

- ■ Breads
- ■ Cereals

IF YOU GET TOO LITTLE

Deficiency of B12 leads to pernicious anemia with symptoms of fatigue, lightheadedness, headache and irritability. Other symptoms may include nausea, loss of appetite, sore mouth, diarrhea, confusion, memory loss and depression.

IF YOU TAKE TOO MUCH

There are no known toxic effects for vitamin B12.

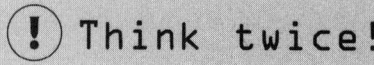

(!) Think twice!

Taking large doses of vitamin B12 can cause a hypersensitivity reaction such as a rash or hives in people with low potassium levels.

(?) Did you know?

Aging is a more common cause of vitamin B12 deficiency than is poor dietary intake. Intrinsic factor slows as you age, which makes it more difficult for your body to absorb the B12 you get from foods or pills.

📄 Startling statistics

If you don't have enough intrinsic factor to absorb vitamin B12 from foods, you probably won't be able to get much from supplements either. Some healthcare providers recommend injections of B12 for strict vegetarians and older people.

KITCHEN CONNECTIONS

✔ *Have a Swiss cheese and tuna melt sandwich.*
✔ *Add scrambled egg pieces to fried rice.*
✔ *Vegans should include fortified cereals with fortified soymilk at breakfast.*

NUTRIENT THIEVES

▶ Exposure to light and heat help destroy vitamin B12 in foods.

 Supplement savvy

Large doses of supplemental vitamin C will decrease the amount of vitamin B12 you can absorb.

As with all B complex vitamins, it's not smart to take individual pills since this family of nutrients works best as a group.

TURKEY DIVAN

So many great sources of vitamin B12 … let's try turkey! Here is an updated and lightened version of the old classic. Nondairy creamer or half-and-half is used instead of heavy whipping cream, and sliced water chestnuts are added to broccoli florets. This dish is elegant enough for guests, but it can also be quickly assembled for the family.

> 1 (14-oz.) bag frozen baby broccoli florets, thawed
> 1 cup sliced water chestnuts
> ¼ cup each margarine, all-purpose flour
> 1½ cups reduced-sodium chicken broth
> ¼ cup half-and-half
> 3 tablespoons sherry or vermouth
> 1 teaspoon Worcestershire sauce
> Dash nutmeg
> 1¼ cups (5 oz.) freshly grated Parmesan cheese
> ¾ lb. cooked sliced turkey
> Dash paprika

1 Heat oven to 425°F.

2 Cook broccoli florets in microwave 6 to 7 minutes on High power; drain well. Transfer to 3-quart casserole. Scatter water chestnuts over broccoli; set aside.

3 In medium saucepan, melt margarine over medium heat; add flour. Let mixture cook while stirring briskly 1 minute.

4 Add broth, whisking constantly until mixture comes to a boil. Cook an additional 1 to 2 minutes or until thickened. Remove from heat. Add half-and-half, sherry, Worcestershire sauce, nutmeg and ¾ cup of the Parmesan cheese. Stir well until smooth.

5 Arrange sliced turkey over vegetables. Pour sauce over vegetables, spreading with spoon to cover. Sprinkle with remaining Parmesan cheese and paprika. Bake 20 to 30 minutes or until internal temperature reaches 180°F and topping is hot and bubbly.

6 servings.
Preparation time: 15 minutes.
Ready to serve: 1 hour, 15 minutes.
Per serving: 340 calories, 19 g fat (7 g saturated fat), 65 mg cholesterol, 825 mg sodium, 2.5 g fiber.

Pantothenic Acid or Vitamin B5

The name pantothenic acid comes from the Greek word pantos, meaning "everywhere," referring to its wide availability in foods. Therefore, it is easily accessible in the diet. Significant amounts of pantothenic acid are lost, though, when foods are refined or heavily processed.

RECOMMENDED INTAKE

AI (Adequate Intake)
Pantothenic Acid (mg/d)

Life-Stage	Children	Men	Women	Pregnancy	Lactation
1-3 years	2				
4-8 years	3				
9-13 years	4			6	7
14-18 years		5	5	6	7
19-30 years		5	5	6	7
31-50 years		5	5	6	7
51-70 years		5	5		
70+ years		5	5		

Source: The National Academy of Sciences

What Is It?

Pantothenic acid, also known as vitamin B5, is a member of the water-soluble B vitamin family. It is an essential ingredient of two substances (coenzyme A and acyl carrier protein), which are needed to metabolize carbohydrates and fats.

Why You Need It

Hormones

Normal adrenal gland function requires pantothenic acid, as it is essential for production of adrenal hormones, such as cortisone, which play an essential part in your body's reaction to stress. Pantothenic acid is also necessary for the production of other steroid hormones and cholesterol, as well as vitamin A, vitamin D and vitamin B12.

Immune System

Antibody synthesis requires pantothenic acid; it is also involved in wound healing.

Metabolism

Pantothenic acid is essential for the release of energy from food. It is used in the manufacture of a compound called coenzyme A, which plays a vital role in the breakdown of fats and carbohydrates. It is also necessary for building cell membranes.

Nervous System & Brain

Pantothenic acid is necessary for the production of some neurotransmitters, such as acetylcholine, and is essential for normal nervous system function.

More or Less?

Increased or decreased nutrient needs should always be discussed with your healthcare professional.

You may need higher than recommended amounts of vitamin B5 if you abuse alcohol.

▶▶ Best natural food sources

- ■ Almost all foods

▶▶ Fortified foods

- ■ Whole grain cereals

If You Get Too Little

Deficiency of this nutrient is extremely rare except in cases of severe, prolonged malnutrition. Symptoms include adrenal gland abnormalities and graying hair.

If You Take Too Much

As with deficiency, toxic levels of B5 are rare. Symptoms include diarrhea, fluid retention, drowsiness and depression.

(!) Think twice!

Long-term use of sulfa drugs, sleeping pills and alcohol may increase your need for pantothenic acid.

(Continued...)

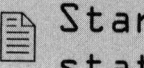 **Did you know?**

There is no Daily Recommended Intake (DRI) for pantothenic acid because deficiency is so rare. The federal government decided to not use scarce resources on determining a DRI for this overly abundant nutrient. Only adequate intakes have been established.

Startling statistics

Vitamin B5 is the only B vitamin not added back to enriched grains. Whole wheat breads and cereals are your best choices.

KITCHEN CONNECTIONS

✔ *Try a whole grain pita with hummus for variety.*
✔ *Eat a variety of fresh vegetables; they contain more pantothenic acid than cooked vegetables.*

NUTRIENT THIEVES

▶ Pantothenic acid is easily destroyed by acids (such as vinegar) or alkalis (such as baking soda) and by dry heat. More than half of the pantothenic acid in wheat is lost during milling, and about one-third is lost in meat during cooking.

 Supplement savvy

Separate supplements of B5 are not needed or recommended. As with all B complex vitamins, it's not smart to take individual pills since this family of nutrients works best as a group.

SOUTHWESTERN HOMINY SOUP

This hearty chili-seasoned soup is a great way to transform leftover chicken or turkey into a distinctive and satisfying meal that, like most foods, offers your body plenty of vitamin B5.

2 teaspoons olive oil or vegetable oil
1 large onion, chopped
1 small red bell pepper, seeded, diced
3 garlic cloves, minced
1 (4-oz.) can diced green chiles
1 tablespoon chili powder
1 teaspoon ground cumin
1 tablespoon chopped fresh oregano
    or 1 teaspoon dried
5 cups reduced-sodium chicken broth
2 (15-oz.) cans white hominy, drained, rinsed
1 (15-oz.) can diced tomatoes, undrained
2 cups diced cooked chicken or turkey
½ cup chopped fresh cilantro
¼ teaspoon freshly ground pepper
Lime wedges

❶ In 4- to 6-quart soup pot, heat oil over medium-high heat until hot. Add onion and bell pepper; cook 3 to 5 minutes or until tender, stirring frequently. Add garlic, green chiles, chili powder, cumin and oregano; cook 30 seconds, stirring constantly. Add broth, hominy and tomatoes; bring to a simmer. Reduce heat to low. Skim off any foam. Simmer, covered, about 20 minutes or until vegetables are tender and flavors have blended.

❷ Add chicken and ¼ cup of the cilantro; simmer 3 to 4 minutes or until heated through. Stir in pepper. Ladle soup into bowls. Garnish with a sprinkling of remaining cilantro. Serve with lime wedges.

10 (1-cup) servings.
Preparation time: 20 minutes.
Ready to serve: 1 hour, 10 minutes.
Per serving: 155 calories, 4 g total fat (1 g saturated fat), 20 mg cholesterol, 575 mg sodium, 3.5 g fiber.

Biotin

B ios is the Greek word for life. Bacteria in the intestines usually produce enough biotin, but it is also widely available in small amounts in most common foods.

WHAT IS IT?

Technically, biotin isn't a true vitamin. It's a nutrient that is synthesized by the bacteria in your intestinal

RECOMMENDED INTAKE

AI (Adequate Intake)

Biotin (mcg/d)

Life-Stage	Children	Men	Women	Pregnancy	Lactation
1-3 years	8				
4-8 years	12				
9-13 years	20			30	35
14-18 years		25	25	30	35
19-30 years		30	30	30	35
31-50 years		30	30	30	35
51-70 years		30	30		
70+ years		30	30		

Source: The National Academy of Sciences

tract. You can make all the biotin you need in your intestines. In fact, most people excrete more biotin in waste products than they take in through foods.

WHY YOU NEED IT

Metabolism
Biotin is needed for carbohydrate metabolism and helps in the synthesis of fatty acids. It also helps join amino acids into proteins.

Skin & Hair
Biotin is important to help keep your hair and nails healthy.

MORE OR LESS?

Increased or decreased nutrient needs should always be discussed with your healthcare professional.

You may need higher than recommended amounts of biotin if you are a:

* *Smoker*
* *Alcohol abuser*
* *Person who eats huge quantities of raw egg whites*
* *Person on long-term anticonvulsant medication therapy*

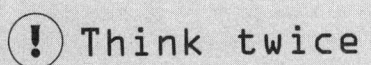

▶▶ Best natural food sources

- ■ Eggs
- ■ Yeast breads

▶▶ Fortified foods

- ■ Ready-to-eat hot and cold cereals

IF YOU GET TOO LITTLE

It's almost impossible to be deficient in biotin because it's made in your intestines. If you eat lots of raw egg whites, you might have symptoms including hair loss, nausea, depression and insomnia. Infants on formulas that are deficient in biotin may develop cradle cap (flaking skin on the head) or have poor muscle tone.

IF YOU TAKE TOO MUCH

No toxic effects have been linked with biotin intake.

(!) Think twice!

Prolonged use of anticonvulsant medications may lead to biotin deficiency.

(?) Did you know?

Biotin was "discovered" three times and is sometimes called coenzyme R or vitamin H.

(Continued...)

81

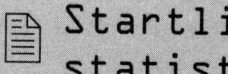 **Startling statistics**

Long-term antibiotic use can kill off intestinal bacteria that you need to make biotin.

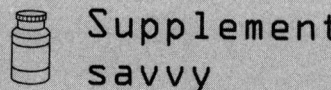 **Supplement savvy**

As with all B complex vitamins, it's not smart to take individual pills since this family of nutrients works best as a group.

KITCHEN CONNECTIONS

✔ *Many foods contain biotin, but most have only small amounts.*

✔ *Mix some brown rice with slivered almonds.*

✔ *Whip up a batch of French toast with an egg and milk batter.*

NUTRIENT THIEVES

▶ The only concern really comes with the consumption of raw eggs. Avidin, a protein and carbohydrate molecule in the egg white, binds with biotin in the stomach and decreases its absorption. Cooking destroys the avidin, so the only concern about this interaction is with raw egg consumption. Otherwise, biotin is one of the most stable of the B vitamins.

COUNTRY-STYLE WHITE LOAVES

Yeast breads feature biotin as a nutrient, so here's an excellent basic loaf you'll love. Be precise about the temperature of the added liquid. This dough may be frozen for up to one month, then baked and enjoyed oven-fresh.

5¼ cups all-purpose flour
2 tablespoons sugar
2 (¼-oz.) pkgs. active dry yeast
1½ teaspoons salt
2 tablespoons butter
1 cup water
1 cup milk

1 In large bowl, combine 2 cups of the flour, sugar, yeast and salt. Set aside. In small saucepan, melt 2 tablespoons butter over medium heat. Add water and milk; heat to 110° to 115°F.

2 In large bowl, combine flour and butter mixtures; beat 2 minutes at high speed. Add another 1 cup flour; beat an additional 1 to 2 minutes at high speed until smooth. With wooden spoon, stir in enough remaining flour to form soft dough. Turn out onto floured surface. Knead 5 to 8 minutes or until dough is smooth and elastic.

3 Place in greased bowl, turning to coat all sides of dough. Cover with kitchen towel and set in warm, draft-free area 45 minutes or until doubled.

4 Heat oven to 400°F. Spray 2 (9x5-inch) loaf pans with nonstick cooking spray.

5 On floured surface, roll one-half of the dough into 12x7-inch rectangle. Beginning with short end, roll up as for jelly roll. Pinch ends to seal, and place, seam side down, in loaf pan. Repeat with remaining dough. Bake 45 minutes or until crust is golden. Remove from pan immediately. Cool on wire rack.

2 loaves.
Preparation time: 1 hour, 30 minutes.
Ready to serve: 2 hours, 45 minutes.
Per serving: 120 calories, 2 g fat (1 g saturated fat), 5 mg cholesterol, 160 mg sodium, 1 g fiber.

Choline

Choline and inositol (page 88) are "unofficial" vitamins. They don't rate full vitamin status because your body manufactures these compounds and you don't have to get them from foods. There are no RDAs or DRIs for these nutrients because almost nobody is ever deficient. Since scientists have spent less time investigating these nutri-ents, less is known about them than the full-fledged vitamins. Of course, that may change with time.

Choline is related to the substance lecithin. In fact, lecithin is a source of choline. Lecithin is not an essential nutrient because your body can make all that it needs. Choline, on the other hand, has been elevated to nutrient status.

RECOMMENDED INTAKE

AI (Adequate Intake)

Choline (mg/d)

Life-Stage	Children	Men	Women	Pregnancy	Lactation
1-3 years	200				
4-8 years	250				
9-13 years	375			450	550
14-18 years		550	400	450	550
19-30 years		550	425	450	550
31-50 years		550	425	450	550
51 70 years		550	425		
70+ years		550	425		

Source: The National Academy of Sciences

WHAT IS IT?

The Food and Nutrition Board recently set a precedent by classifying choline as a nutrient, even though it's not essential for all people. Research suggests that men and pregnant or breast-feeding women require a dietary source of choline of 500 mg per day. These three groups have the highest calorie needs and may not be able to make enough of this nutrient in the liver.

WHY YOU NEED IT

Choline helps your brain store memories and keeps your emotions and judgment in line. This vitamin-like compound works as a precursor to the nerve messenger acetylcholine and helps maintain smooth, fluid connections between brain cells. Small quantities are made in your liver with the help of vitamin B12, folic acid and methionine. It's thought that higher amounts than your body makes are required for optimal health. Pregnant women have lots of choline circulating around the placenta. That's the organ that passes nutrients from the mother to the developing baby. It's been suggested, but not proven, that choline is important for fetal growth.

▶▶ Best natural food sources

- Brewer's yeast
- Eggs
- Legumes
- Meat
- Nuts
- Whole grains

▶▶ Fortified foods

- None

IF YOU GET TOO LITTLE

There are no known deficiency symptoms for choline. Most people consume between 300 to 1,000 mg per day from foods.

IF YOU TAKE TOO MUCH

Taking more than 10 grams of choline per day may give you an unpleasant fishy body odor.

(!) Think twice!

DMAE is a chemical similar to choline, but there is scant research on its effects when taken as a dietary supplement.

(?) Did you know?

People with Alzheimer's disease often have unusually low brain levels of acetylcholine. Plenty of research is underway to explore this fact, but there's no evidence yet that supplemental choline would be beneficial.

(Continued...)

NUTRIENT THIEVES

▶ Choline is sensitive to water and may be destroyed by cooking, food processing or improper food storage (that is, exposure to oxygen).

 Supplement savvy

Lecithin is the most common source of choline in supplements and provides approximately 10 to 20 percent of its weight as choline. This fat-like compound spoils quickly—keep it refrigerated.

CANNELLINI BEAN, CHICKEN & PESTO SALAD

The beans (legumes) and chicken provide choline in this quick-and-easy Italian main dish salad. If you're counting calories, go light on the pesto.

1½ lbs. boneless skinless chicken breasts,
   rinsed, cut into ½-inch strips
½ cup olive oil
2 garlic cloves, minced
½ teaspoon salt
1 small onion, minced
4 tablespoons prepared pesto
1 tablespoon white wine vinegar
2 (15-oz.) cans cannellini beans, drained, rinsed*
Chopped fresh basil or flat-leaf parsley

1 In large bowl, combine chicken with 2 tablespoons olive oil, garlic, salt and onion; toss to coat chicken well. Cover and refrigerate 4 hours.

2 In heavy nonstick skillet, heat 1 tablespoon oil over high heat until hot. Add chicken and cook about 5 minutes, tossing with wooden spatula until chicken is no longer pink in center.

3 In medium bowl, combine pesto with remaining oil, vinegar, chicken and cannellini beans. Garnish with basil or parsley.

TIP *Cannellini beans are white beans used in Italian cooking; they are the same size and shape as kidney beans. You can substitute navy beans but cannellini beans are softer.

4 to 6 servings.
Preparation time: 10 minutes.
Ready to serve: 4 hours, 10 minutes.
Per serving: 705 calories, 37 g total fat (6.5 g saturated fat), 95.5 mg cholesterol, 570 mg sodium, 11 g fiber.

Inositol

Inositol and choline (page 84) are "unofficial" vitamins. They don't rate full vitamin status because your body manufactures these compounds and you don't have to get them from foods. There are no RDAs or DRIs for these nutrients because almost nobody is ever deficient. Since scientists have spent less time investigating these nutrients, less is known about them than the full-fledged vitamins. Of course, that may change with time.

WHAT IS IT?

Inositol is a major component of the fat-like substance lecithin. Like choline, it promotes the removal of fat from the liver. Inositol also is involved in the control of blood cholesterol levels. Your intestinal bacteria can make inositol in limited amounts, and no deficiency diseases have been reported.

WHY YOU NEED IT

Inositol keeps cell membranes healthy and shuttles needed fat from place to place. It also helps keep your bone marrow, eye tissue and intestines in good condition.

RECOMMENDED INTAKE

There is no RDA or AI established for inositol. Most people consume about 1,000 mg from foods each day.

▶▶ Best natural food sources

- Inositol is found in a wide variety of foods, especially citrus fruits, nuts, beans and whole grains. In plant foods, it is located in the fiber component. In animal foods, it is found primarily in organ meats.

▶▶ Fortified foods

- None

IF YOU GET TOO LITTLE

No deficiency symptoms have ever been reported in humans. In some animal experiments, low levels of inositol have led to fatty livers, nerve disorders and intestinal problems.

IF YOU TAKE TOO MUCH

There have been no reported toxic effects of too much inositol.

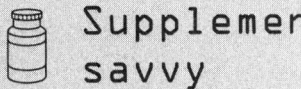

Supplement savvy

Like choline, inositol is found in lecithin supplements, but amounts may vary widely.

? Did you know?

There is no scientific evidence that supplemental inositol helps with any health problem. Current research is evaluating its effect on depression and nerve damage in diabetics.

Minerals

P eople are surprised to learn that up to five pounds of minerals are stored in a human body. Because minerals are critical to proper metabolism and so many functions, you need to understand which minerals are necessary, how they help you, and how to get enough of them (but not too much). This chapter will help in that regard, making sure the 100 daily milligrams of minerals you need are the right ones.

How to Use This Chapter

Each mineral is described in a variety of ways:

What Is It?
A brief description of each mineral.

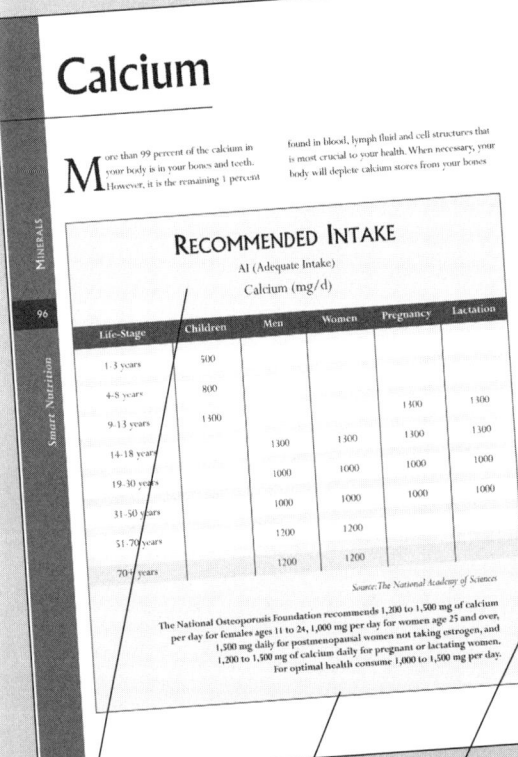

Recommended Intake
These are the highest current recommendations based on federal guidelines.

Optimal Intake
These levels might be higher than the current RDA or DV (defined on page 20). Optimal intake amounts are based on the analysis of scientific studies, review papers and interviews with leading experts.

Why You Need It
This section summarizes the main functions of the mineral based on the following classifications:

- Antioxidant Actions
- Bones & Teeth
- Energy Production
- Hormonal Balance
- Immune System
- Metabolism
- Nervous System & Brain
- Skin & Hair
- Other

Best Natural Food Sources
These are foods that provide at least 25 percent of the RDA in just one serving. If you are low in any particular mineral, scan this list for quick, concentrated food ideas. Liver or organ meats were purposely omitted from these lists, even though they might be excellent vitamin or mineral sources, because an animal's liver is also its toxic waste dump. The risk of harm from consuming toxic substances far outweighs the benefit of concentrated nutrients.

Fortified Foods
Instead of relying on fortified foods, eat foods naturally high in nutrients. Nature's combination of nutrients helps your body absorb and utilize vitamins and minerals. A product fortified with one or more nutrients will not provide the complex package of compounds found in food. Eating fortified foods is a second-rate choice.

More or Less?
Individual differences such as lifestyle, chronic disease status and other factors can increase or decrease your need for a particular mineral. Use this section as a starting point to discuss individual needs with your healthcare provider. Never take more or less than the recommended or optimal amounts of any nutrient without professional guidance.

If You Get Too Little
Common symptoms of low intakes are described, as are the full-blown symptoms of a deficiency disease.

Did You Know?
With so many myths and miscommunications about the value and use of supplements, it's easy to become confused. Common questions or concerns are addressed here to help you separate fact from fiction.

Kitchen Connections
This information will help you learn to make smart food choices and preserve minerals in foods that you store and prepare at home.

Supplement Savvy
If you must take a supplement, here are the facts to help you make an informed choice.

IF YOU GET TOO LITTLE
Too little calcium stunts the development of bones and teeth. A lack of vitamin D, which is needed to absorb calcium, can have the same result. Without enough calcium, your bones soften; this is called rickets in children and osteomalacia in adults. Mild calcium deficiency can cause nerve sensitivity, muscle twitches, irritability, heart palpitations and insomnia.

IF YOU TAKE TOO MUCH
Too much supplemental calcium may cause nausea, vomiting, low blood pressure, irregular heartbeat, kidney stones and impaired absorption of iron, zinc and magnesium. The minimum toxic dose of calcium is 2,500 mg per day.

(!) Think twice!
Excess calcium may decrease the effectiveness of the following medications:

- Digitalis—a heart medicine
- Phenytoin—(Dilantin)—used for seizures
- Tetracycline—a medicine for infections

Do not use bonemeal, dolomite or oyster shell as a source of calcium. The FDA has issued warnings that these products could be contaminated with heavy metals, including lead.

(?) Did you know?
The calcium in soymilk is absorbed 25 percent less efficiently than the calcium in cow's milk. If you rely on soymilk as your primary source of calcium, you should consume at least 25 percent more than the amount listed on the nutrition facts panel to achieve the equivalent of dairy products.

Startling statistics
More women die each year from hip fractures related to osteoporosis than from breast cancer, uterine cancer and ovarian cancer combined.

KITCHEN CONNECTIONS
- Add some tofu to a yogurt smoothie
- Have molasses or almond cookies with a glass of milk
- Top a pizza with Swiss, jack or goat cheese
- Toss broccoli and fresh soybeans in a salad

NUTRIENT THIEVES
There are components of other foods that can reduce calcium absorption. Foods that are high in oxalic acid—such as spinach, rhubarb, chard and chocolate—can interfere with calcium absorption. Phytic acid, or phytates, found in whole grain foods or foods rich in fiber, may reduce the absorption of calcium and other minerals as well.

If you consume a lot of high-protein foods and/or soft drinks, which have lots of phosphorus, you will also need more calcium in the rest of your diet.

Supplement savvy
All calcium supplements don't provide equal amounts of absorbable calcium. The lower the absorption rate, the more you need to take to get an adequate supply.

Type of Calcium	% Absorption
Calcium citrate	74
Calcium carbonate	40
Calcium phosphate	32
Calcium lactate	18
Calcium gluconate	9

Source: Adapted from the Journal of Bone Mineral Research.

Think Twice!
Warning notices for potential interactions are noted here.

If You Take Too Much
The key word here is *take*. It's almost impossible to get too much of a mineral from foods. Misuse of supplements is almost always the reason for the side effects listed. The minimum toxic dose is given, when known. This is the smallest amount of a nutrient that can cause side effects ranging from annoying to life threatening.

Startling Statistics
These will help you put things into perspective.

Nutrient Thieves
This information will help you identify those things that destroy or rob your foods of minerals. You'll also learn how to prevent loss of nutrients.

Boron

Boron is an essential element for plants and now there is evidence that it is also necessary for humans.

WHAT IS IT?

This trace mineral was thought to be essential only for plant foods until recently. Boron is distributed throughout your body with the highest concentrations in bones and tooth enamel. Not identified as an essential nutrient until 1980, the functions of boron are not completely known.

WHY YOU NEED IT

Bones & Teeth
Because boron works with calcium, magnesium and phosphorus, it is thought to play a role in the formation of bone tissue.

Hormones
Boron affects the metabolism of steroid hormones and may also have a role in converting vitamin D to its more active form. Boron also may play a role in male sex hormone production.

RECOMMENDED INTAKE

There is no RDA or AI developed yet for boron. Most people get 2 to 5 mg per day from foods, and that appears to be adequate.

MORE OR LESS?

Increased or decreased nutrient needs should always be discussed with your healthcare professional.

You may need higher than recommended amounts of boron if you are at risk for osteoporosis.

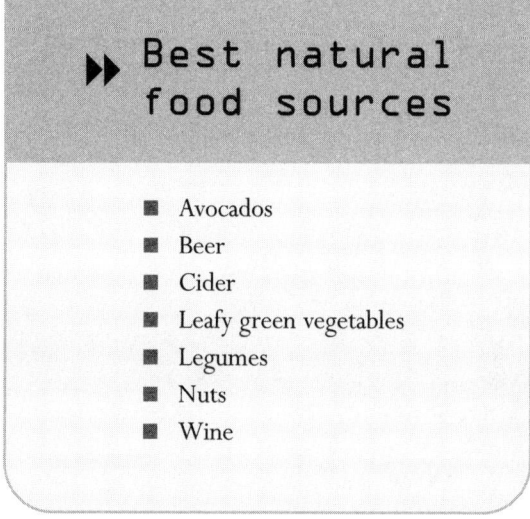

▶▶ Best natural food sources

- Avocados
- Beer
- Cider
- Leafy green vegetables
- Legumes
- Nuts
- Wine

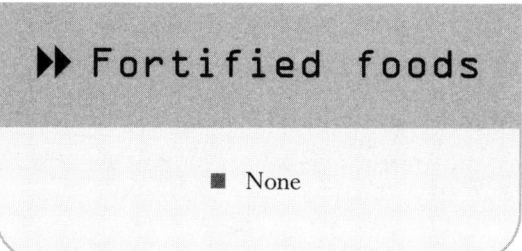

▶▶ Fortified foods

- None

IF YOU GET TOO LITTLE

There is not enough experience or research with this element to know what the signs of deficiency might be, though poor bone development is a logical consequence.

IF YOU TAKE TOO MUCH

It's very hard to take too much boron, since it's not commonly found on supplement shelves. Taking borax products may cause toxicity with symptoms such as poor appetite, nausea, vomiting, diarrhea and fatigue. A minimum toxic dose has not been established, but 18 to 20 grams in a single dose have caused death in adults.

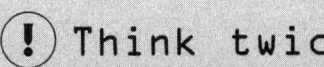 **Think twice!**

Boron can affect hormone levels and should not be supplemented in those at risk for prostate, breast or other hormone-related cancers.

Borax or boron-containing powders should never be applied to mucous membranes or applied to open wounds since this element is readily absorbed and toxic effects can occur.

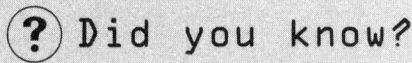 **Did you know?**

There may be a link between boron and osteoarthritis. Epidemiological studies show countries where boron is low tend to have a higher incidence of osteoarthritis compared to countries where boron intake is relatively high. It's too soon to draw any conclusions.

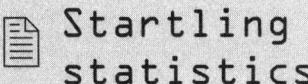 **Startling statistics**

Though coffee and milk are fairly low in boron, they make up about 12 percent of the average daily intake, simply because of the volume of these beverages commonly consumed.

KITCHEN CONNECTIONS

✔ *If you have hard water, it may be rich in boron.*

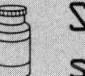 **Supplement savvy**

Take boron only as part of a multivitamin and mineral supplement that provides no more than 3 mg per day.

Calcium

M ore than 99 percent of the calcium in your body is in your bones and teeth. However, it is the remaining 1 percent found in blood, lymph fluid and cell structures that is most crucial to your health. When necessary, your body will deplete calcium stores from your bones

RECOMMENDED INTAKE

AI (Adequate Intake)
Calcium (mg/d)

Life-Stage	Children	Men	Women	Pregnancy	Lactation
1-3 years	500				
4-8 years	800				
9-13 years	1300			1300	1300
14-18 years		1300	1300	1300	1300
19-30 years		1000	1000	1000	1000
31-50 years		1000	1000	1000	1000
51-70 years		1200	1200		
70+ years		1200	1200		

Source: The National Academy of Sciences

The National Osteoporosis Foundation recommends 1,200 to 1,500 mg of calcium per day for females ages 11 to 24, 1,000 mg per day for women age 25 and over, 1,500 mg daily for postmenopausal women not taking estrogen, and 1,200 to 1,500 mg of calcium daily for pregnant or lactating women. For optimal health consume 1,000 to 1,500 mg per day.

and weaken them to provide blood calcium levels required for circulation, nerve transmission and muscle contraction.

WHAT IS IT?

The white powdery mineral that you can see in chalk, ivory and pearls is calcium. It accounts for about 3½ pounds of weight in an adult male and approximately 2¼ pounds in the average female. Calcium absorption will vary widely over your life-span. Infants absorb about 60 percent of the calcium they take in; following infancy, absorption rates decline dramatically. During puberty, calcium absorption rebounds and then levels off at about 25 percent in early adulthood. Calcium absorption gradually declines with age at about the rate of .2 percent a year for postmenopausal women and older men.

WHY YOU NEED IT

Bones & Teeth
Bone is living, growing tissue that is constantly being broken down and rebuilt, just like your hair and nails. About 20 percent of your skeleton is made brand new every year. Calcium intake is critical because it's the most abundant mineral in your body. Since blood levels of calcium are your body's priority, blood tests are not a good indicator of your calcium status. Bone density tests are the best way to measure the strength of your skeletal system.

Cardiovascular System
Calcium assists in muscle contraction, blood clotting and maintenance of cell membranes. It's also critical for heartbeat regulation through its effects on the heart muscle.

Nervous System & Brain
Calcium is essential for nerve impulse conduction. It also plays a role in the release of neurotransmitters and activates some enzymes that help generate nerve impulses.

MORE OR LESS?

Increased or decreased nutrient needs should always be discussed with your healthcare professional.

You may need higher than recommended amounts of calcium if you:
- *Avoid milk*
- *Are on a very low-calorie diet*
- *Eat lots of high-protein foods*
- *Are postmenopausal*
- *Are age 9 to 19*

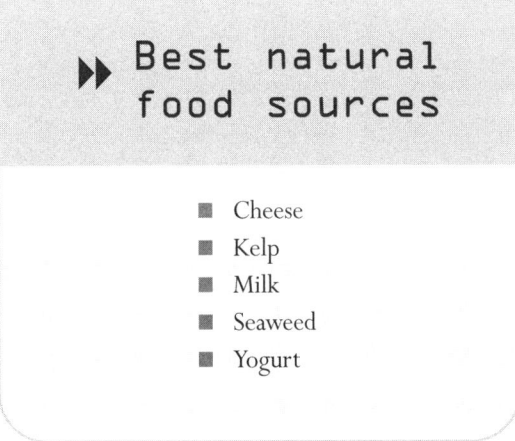

▶▶ Best natural food sources

- ■ Cheese
- ■ Kelp
- ■ Milk
- ■ Seaweed
- ■ Yogurt

▶▶ Fortified foods

- ■ Some kinds of orange juice
- ■ Some kinds of rice
- ■ Tofu (made with calcium sulfate)

(Continued...)

IF YOU GET TOO LITTLE

Too little calcium stunts the development of bones and teeth. A lack of vitamin D, which is needed to absorb calcium, can have the same result. Without enough calcium, your bones soften; this is called rickets in children and osteomalacia in adults. Mild calcium deficiency can cause nerve sensitivity, muscle twitches, irritability, heart palpitations and insomnia.

IF YOU TAKE TOO MUCH

Too much supplemental calcium may cause nausea, vomiting, low blood pressure, irregular heartbeat, kidney stones and impaired absorption of iron, zinc and magnesium. The minimum toxic dose of calcium is 2,500 mg per day.

 Think twice!

Excess calcium may decrease the effectiveness of the following medications:

• Digitalis—a heart medicine
• Phenytoin—(Dilantin)—used for seizures
• Tetracycline—a medicine for infections

Do not use bonemeal, dolomite or oyster shell as a source of calcium. The FDA has issued warnings that these products could be contaminated with heavy metals, including lead.

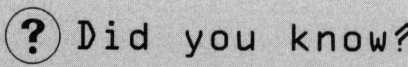 Did you know?

The calcium in soymilk is absorbed 25 percent less efficiently than the calcium in cow's milk. If you rely on soymilk as your primary source of calcium, you should consume at least 25 percent more than the amount listed on the nutrition facts panel to achieve the equivalent of dairy products.

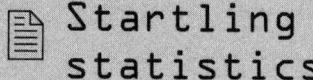 Startling statistics

More women die each year from hip fractures related to osteoporosis than from breast cancer, uterine cancer and ovarian cancer combined.

Kitchen Connections

- ✔ *Add some tofu to a yogurt smoothie.*
- ✔ *Have molasses or almond cookies with a glass of milk.*
- ✔ *Top a pizza with Swiss, jack or goat cheese.*
- ✔ *Toss broccoli and fresh soybeans in a salad.*

Nutrient Thieves

▶ There are components of other foods that can reduce calcium absorption. Foods that are high in oxalic acid—such as spinach, rhubarb, chard and chocolate—can interfere with calcium absorption. Phytic acid, or phytates, found in whole grain foods or foods rich in fiber, may reduce the absorption of calcium and other minerals as well.

If you consume a lot of high-protein foods and/or soft drinks, which have lots of phosphorus, you will also need more calcium in the rest of your diet.

 Supplement savvy

All calcium supplements don't provide equal amounts of absorbable calcium. The lower the absorption rate, the more you need to take to get an adequate supply.

Type of Calcium	% Absorption
Calcium citrate	74
Calcium carbonate	40
Calcium phosphate	32
Calcium lactate	18
Calcium gluconate	9

Source: Adapted from the Journal of Bone Mineral Research.

Chloride

You may not know much about chloride alone, but it's part of a famous couple known as table salt (sodium chloride). Adults typically need a minimum of 750 mg of chloride a day. Part of that goes to form hydrochloric acid—better known as stomach acid. This caustic compound is what helps you break down food so individual nutrients can be absorbed and used by the body.

What Is It?

Chloride is an electrolyte that helps maintain the balance of water between body cells and surrounding fluids. Chloride is the negative ion that helps neutralize the positively charged sodium and potassium ions within cells. You have about 4 teaspoons of chloride in your body.

Why You Need It

Fluid Balance

Chloride ions located mainly outside cell walls help monitor and regulate the flow of fluid inside and outside cell walls. Excess chloride is removed through sweat, urine and feces.

Metabolism

Chloride combines with hydrogen to make hydrochloric acid, which helps nutrient absorption during digestion.

Nervous System & Brain

Transmission of nerve impulses to the brain and regulation of electrical impulses that travel across nerves are aided by chloride.

Recommended Intake

There is no RDA or AI established for chloride. Most experts suggest about 750 mg per day (the amount found in ¼ teaspoon of table salt), or more if you exercise.

More or Less?

Increased or decreased nutrient needs should always be discussed with your healthcare professional.

You may need higher than recommended amounts of chloride if you:
* *Have been profusely sweating for a long period of time*
* *Have chronic diarrhea or vomiting*

▶▶ Best natural food sources

- Salted foods
- Table salt

▶▶ Fortified foods

- None

IF YOU GET TOO LITTLE

Alkalosis, or too little chloride, is rare. Alkalosis can occur with excessive sweat loss or with prolonged diarrhea or vomiting. Symptoms include muscle weakness, loss of appetite and lethargy.

IF YOU TAKE TOO MUCH

Too much chloride is rare and only likely if you are consuming huge amounts of salt or salt substitutes that contain potassium chloride. Overdose may cause weakness, confusion, increased blood pressure or coma.

 Supplement savvy

Chloride supplements are not generally available, nor is chloride found in multivitamin/mineral supplements. Only people with Bartter's syndrome or those who vomit frequently should ever take extra chloride under the direction and supervision of their healthcare provider.

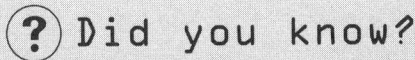 ? Did you know?

When you sweat, you lose not only sodium, but chloride, too. Fortunately, foods that contain sodium usually contain chloride as well.

Chromium

The mineral chromium is the same stuff that makes old-fashioned car bumpers shiny. It also helps you shine when you need to work or play hard. Because it helps regulate insulin, chromium is important in helping you maintain peak energy under pressure. That doesn't mean it will make you stronger, smarter or capable of more than is normal for you.

WHAT IS IT?

Researchers discovered that the mineral chromium

RECOMMENDED INTAKE

AI (Adequate Intake)

Chromium (mcg/d)

Life-Stage	Children	Men	Women	Pregnancy	Lactation
1-3 years	11				
4-8 years	15				
9-13 years		25	21	29	44
14-18 years		35	24	29	44
19-30 years		35	25	30	45
31-50 years		35	25	30	45
51-70 years		30	20		
70+ years		30	20		

Source: The National Academy of Sciences

For optimal health consume 50 to 200 mcg per day.

in the trivalent form—chromium that's combined with three hydrogen atoms or in which three hydrogen atoms are replaced—is one of the major components of glucose tolerance factor (GTF). The effects of chromium were first identified in 1955 when researchers found that feeding brewer's yeast to glucose-intolerant rats resulted in normal glucose tolerance, the ability of cells to take up glucose for energy use. This previously unknown connection established chromium as an essential trace nutrient. This mineral is stored in your brain, skin, fat, muscles, spleen, kidneys and testes.

WHY YOU NEED IT

Metabolism
Chromium works with insulin to help your body use glucose and maintain normal blood sugar levels. We still don't fully understand the role of chromium other than knowing that it is somehow involved with protein, fat and carbohydrate metabolism.

MORE OR LESS?

Increased or decreased nutrient needs should always be discussed with your healthcare professional.

You may need higher than recommended amounts of chromium if you are:

- *Age 70 or older*
- *Recovering from surgery*
- *A type 2 diabetic*

▶▶ Best natural food sources

- Apples
- Beef
- Brewer's yeast
- Corn on the cob
- Eggs
- Prunes
- Soy flour
- Sweet potatoes
- Wheat germ or bran

▶▶ Fortified foods

- None

IF YOU GET TOO LITTLE

Borderline chromium deficiency is thought to be common—especially in older people. There seems to be a connection between chromium deficiency and the risk of diabetes increasing as you age. It might be linked to the fact that diets high in simple sugars tend to increase chromium losses. But that doesn't mean that high sugar diets cause diabetes. Almost all adult-onset diabetes is caused by weight gain. Getting adequate amounts of chromium may decrease insulin injection doses and improve how certain diabetics handle glucose. Common symptoms of deficiency include depression, confusion, weight loss, increased thirst and weakness.

(Continued...)

IF YOU TAKE TOO MUCH

Athletes who supplement with chromium picolinate are prone to dehydration. Early studies indicate that prolonged over-supplementation with chromium can lead to chronic disease of the kidneys or liver. Long-term environmental exposure from electro-plating, steel manufacturing, cement manufacturing, glass and jewelry making, photography, textile dyeing and wood preserving may cause skin problems, liver and kidney damage, and cancer.

 Think twice!

Antacids can reduce chromium absorption.

(?) Did you know?

There is no scientific evidence that chromium picolinate has any effect on weight loss.

Foods high in simple carbohydrates, like refined grains and sugars, are usually low in chromium and cause your body to lose additional chromium too.

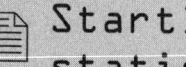 **Startling statistics**

Yeast GFT, not chromium picolinate, is the most biologically active form of chromium and is found in brewster's yeast.

KITCHEN CONNECTIONS

✔ *Add 1 to 2 tablespoons of brewer's yeast or wheat germ to your favorite cookie dough before baking.*
✔ *Grab some tap water! Hard water often contains some chromium; it may supply up to half your daily needs.*
✔ *Make breakfast burritos with whole-wheat tortillas, chopped chiles and eggs.*
✔ *Cook acidic foods (like tomato sauce) in stainless steel pots. Tiny amounts of chromium will be absorbed into the food and add to your dietary intake.*

NUTRIENT THIEVES

▶ Limit refined and highly processed foods since most of the chromium is lost during food processing.

 Supplement savvy

Most multivitamin/mineral supplements contain some chromium.

Individual supplementation with chromium is not recommended.

BEEF BRISKET WITH ROOT VEGETABLES

Here's a robust winter dinner dish that's easy to serve and tender enough to cut with a fork. It's perfect for a buffet or holiday table, or for dividing leftovers into family or single-size containers to freeze. The beef and vegetables, of course, are full of vitamins and minerals you need.

1 tablespoon all-purpose flour
1 (4-lb.) first cut brisket, trimmed
1 cup meatless marinara sauce
½ cup beer
3 bay leaves
3 medium onions, quartered
3 large carrots, cut into 1-inch pieces
2 large potatoes, cut into 1½-inch pieces
1 large parsnip, sliced ½ inch thick
6 garlic cloves, halved
⅛ teaspoon salt
⅛ teaspoon freshly ground pepper

1 Heat oven to 325°F. Dust inside of large roasting bag with flour; set in roasting pan. Place brisket in bag.

2 In large bowl, combine marinara sauce, beer and bay leaves; mix well. Pour over meat, tilting bag to coat underside of meat.

3 Arrange onions, carrots, potatoes, parsnip and garlic around meat, spooning some of the marinara mixture over vegetables.

4 Tie bag closed. Cut 3 or 4 (½-inch) slits into bag.

5 Cook 2½ to 3 hours or until internal temperature reaches at least 160°F.

6 Let rest 15 minutes before slicing. Discard bay leaves. Arrange sliced brisket and vegetables on warm platter.

7 Skim fat from pan juices. Season with salt and pepper. Drizzle juices over brisket. Pour remainder into warm gravy boat and pass.

8 to 10 servings.
Preparation time: 25 minutes.
Ready to serve: 3 hours, 45 minutes.
Per serving: 655 calories, 43 g fat (17 g saturated fat), 135 mg cholesterol, 291 mg sodium, 4 g fiber.

Copper

The amount of copper found in the human body would probably fit on the head of a pin. But such a tiny quantity doesn't prevent this mighty mineral from performing some impressive feats to promote optimal health. In January 2001, the National Academy of Sciences issued the first RDA for copper as a benchmark for ensuring adequate intake.

WHAT IS IT?

Copper is a brownish red metallic element usually

RECOMMENDED INTAKE

RDA (Recommended Dietary Allowance)
Copper (mcg/d)

Life-Stage	Children	Men	Women	Pregnancy	Lactation
1-3 years	340				
4-8 years	440				
9-13 years	700			1000	1300
14-18 years		890	890	1000	1300
19-30 years		900	900	1000	1300
31-50 years		900	900	1000	1300
51-70 years		900	900		
70+ years		900	900		

Source: The National Academy of Sciences

For optimal health consume 2 to 3 mg per day.

found in foods containing iron. As part of at least 13 enzymes, copper is crucial to a variety of functions. Your liver and brain contain the largest amounts of copper, while small amounts are stored in other organs.

WHY YOU NEED IT

Antioxidant Action
Copper is part of the copper-zinc team that helps protect against damage by free radicals.

Bones & Teeth
Bones, joints and connective tissues require copper to help jump-start enzymes that make and maintain these structures.

Nervous System & Brain
Copper is used to make cell membranes and maintains the protective covering around nerve cells.

Skin & Hair
The formation of melanin, a natural coloring pigment in your skin and hair, needs a copper-dependent enzyme.

MORE OR LESS?

Increased or decreased nutrient needs should always be discussed with your healthcare professional.

You may need higher than recommended amounts of copper if you are:
- *A premature infant*
- *Diagnosed with Menkes disease—a genetic disorder that causes copper deficiency*
- *Recovering from severe body burns*

You may need lower than recommended amounts of copper if you have:
- *Wilson's disease—a genetic disorder that prevents excretion of copper*

▶▶ Best natural food sources

- ■ Barley
- ■ Crab
- ■ Lobster
- ■ Oysters

▶▶ Fortified foods

- ■ None

IF YOU GET TOO LITTLE

Infants and children on very limited diets are at high risk for copper deficiency. Symptoms in children include failure to thrive, pale skin tone, diarrhea, lack of pigment in hair and obviously dilated veins. Adult deficiency symptoms are water retention, irritability, poor hair texture and color and a loss of the sense of taste.

IF YOU TAKE TOO MUCH

Symptoms of excess copper include bloody vomit, blood in the urine, dizziness, fainting, severe headache, metallic taste, muscle aches, nausea, liver damage and coma. Wilson's disease, an inherited disorder, causes excess copper accumulation in body tissues. Treatment requires a low-copper diet and medication to bind copper before it can be absorbed. Minimum toxic dose is 20 mg.

(Continued...)

(!) Think twice!

Copper and zinc compete with each other, but not at the levels included in multivitamins. However, if you take a separate zinc supplement, be sure also to take copper. Most experts recommend a ratio of 10 parts zinc to 1 part copper. That means if you take 20 mg of zinc, then you should also take 2 mg of copper.

Supplement savvy

Check your multivitamin/mineral supplement label. If iron and zinc are included (and they should be), make sure copper is listed too.

(?) Did you know?

If your water pipes are made of copper, you're in luck. Drinking water that runs through copper pipes may add a significant amount of this hard-to-get mineral to your intake.

KITCHEN CONNECTIONS

✔ *Using copper pots and pans adds tiny traces of copper to your food intake.*

✔ *Add prunes and buckwheat to oatmeal.*

✔ *Add shrimp and almonds to pasta or stir-fry.*

NUTRIENT THIEVES

▶ Watch out for zinc-rich supplements (especially those popular zinc lozenges). Zinc competes with copper for absorption!

CORN & BARLEY SALAD

If you want to get some copper, barley does the job. More commonly used in soups and breads, barley makes a delicious and healthy addition to this main dish salad.

⅔ cup barley
2 cups cooked corn kernels
1 red bell pepper, cut into ½-inch pieces
¼ cup chopped green onions
¼ cup extra-virgin olive oil
2 teaspoons grated lime zest
2 tablespoons freshly squeezed lime juice
1 tablespoon chopped fresh cilantro
½ teaspoon ground cumin
½ teaspoon garlic salt
½ teaspoon salt
⅛ teaspoon hot pepper sauce

1 Cook barley according to package directions. Let cool.

2 In large bowl, combine barley, corn, bell pepper and onions. In small bowl, whisk together oil, lime zest, lime juice, cilantro, cumin, salts and hot pepper sauce. Pour over barley mixture; toss to coat. Chill several hours to allow flavors to blend.

4 main dish or 6 side dish servings.

Preparation time: 20 minutes.

Ready to serve: 3 hours, 30 minutes.

Per main dish serving: 345 calories, 14.5 g total fat (2 g saturated fat), 0 mg cholesterol, 480 mg sodium, 9 g fiber.

Fluoride

The biggest source of fluoride is usually the local water supply. Half of all United States water supplies are fluoridated. Those that aren't are in homes that rely on well water or non-municipal water sources. Most bottled water does not contain fluoride. Low doses of fluoride are ben-eficial to the dental health of adults as well as children.

If you don't know whether your water is fluori-dated, call your local water department to find out. A typical amount added is .7 to 1.2 mg per liter of water. The American Academy of Pediatrics recom-

RECOMMENDED INTAKE
AI (Adequate Intake)
Fluoride (mg/d)

Life-Stage	Children	Men	Women	Pregnancy	Lactation
1-3 years	0.7				
4-8 years	1				
9-13 years	2			3	3
14-18 years		3	3	3	3
19-30 years		4	3	3	3
31-50 years		4	3	3	3
51-70 years		4	3		
70+ years		4	3		

Source: The National Academy of Sciences

For optimal health consume 1.5 to 4 mg per day.

mends that all breast-fed infants and babies using reconstituted formula in households where the water is not fluoridated start supplements at six months.

WHAT IS IT?

Many experts recommend continuing with supplements until age 16, especially if you drink and cook exclusively with unfluoridated tap or bottled water. Unlike most nutrient supplements, fluoride is only available by prescription from your doctor or dentist.

Fluoride mouth rinses are also available for adults and children over the age of six. The American Dental Association's Council on Dental Therapeutics recommends the use of fluoride by children up to 13 years of age; the American Academy of Pediatrics recommends fluoride supplementation by children until the age of 16 years of age. The 1 mg/5 mL strength rinse is not recommended for use as a supplement by children younger than 6 years of age. Use fluoride rinses immediately after brushing or flossing, just prior to sleep to obtain the maximum protective effect.

WHY YOU NEED IT

Bones & Teeth
Fluoride helps to harden tooth enamel, protects teeth from decay and strengthens all bone tissues.

MORE OR LESS?

Increased or decreased nutrient needs should always be discussed with your healthcare professional.

You may need higher than recommended amounts of fluoride if you have Paget's disease.

▶▶ Best natural food sources

- Not widely found in foods and varies with soil content where foods are grown

▶▶ Fortified foods

- Some municipal drinking water (check with your local water supplier)

IF YOU GET TOO LITTLE

Do you have a mouthful of gleaming silver fillings proving you grew up without benefit of fluoridated water? For more than 60 years, the dental benefits of fluoride have been known. If you drank fluoridated water as a child, you probably have 50 to 70 percent fewer cavities than your peers who didn't have fluoride.

IF YOU TAKE TOO MUCH

Taking 10 mg or more may cause stomach cramps, vomiting, diarrhea and tremors. Long-term high doses cause mottled teeth, brittle bones and increased frequency of broken bones.

(Continued...)

⚠ Think twice!

Toothpaste with fluoride should be spit out and not swallowed; only use a pea-sized amount for children.

? Did you know?

Some bottled water companies and baby food manufacturers now make fluoridated versions of their products.

📄 Startling statistics

Fluoridated drinking water reduces cavities in children by 20 to 40 percent and by 15 to 30 percent in adults. This effect is even greater if you also use fluoridated toothpaste.

KITCHEN CONNECTIONS

✔ *Make juice, soups and stews with fluoridated tap water to be sure your family's teeth are protected.*

Supplement savvy

You may have to go to a dentist to obtain a prescription for fluoride supplements for your breast-fed infant.

WILD RICE & MUSHROOM SOUP

Except for a little too much sodium (and using reduced-sodium chicken broth will fix that!), here's an awfully healthy version of comforting wild rice soup. You'll probably get your fluoride elsewhere, but the mushrooms might provide some!

1 (1-oz.) pkg. dried wild mushrooms
1 cup very hot water (115° to 120°F)
1 tablespoon vegetable oil
1 cup diced pancetta
¼ cup chopped shallots or green onions
1 (8-oz.) pkg. mushrooms, sliced
⅓ cup all-purpose flour
2 cups milk
1 (14.5-oz.) can chicken broth (or an additional
    2 cups milk plus ¾ teaspoon salt)
2 cups cooked wild rice*

❶ Soak dried mushrooms in very hot water in medium bowl 30 minutes. Remove mushrooms; chop. Strain soaking liquid through coffee filter to remove grit; set aside.

❷ Heat oil in Dutch oven over medium-high heat until hot. Add pancetta; sauté 1 minute. Add shallots; sauté 3 to 5 minutes or until tender and pancetta is browned. Add mushrooms; sauté 5 to 8 minutes or until tender. Add chopped wild mushrooms and reserved soaking liquid. Cook 5 minutes or until all liquid is absorbed. Stir in flour; whisk in milk and broth. Bring to a boil; continue cooking, stirring, for several minutes to thicken. Stir in rice; reduce heat to low; simmer 5 minutes.

TIP *To cook wild rice, rinse ¾ cup wild rice under cold water. Place in medium saucepan with 2½ cups water. Add ¾ teaspoon salt. Bring to a boil over medium-high heat. Reduce heat to low; cover and cook 45 to 60 minutes or until grains have opened and rice is chewy-tender. Drain if necessary.

4 main course or 6 first course servings.
Preparation time: 30 minutes.
Ready to serve: 1 hour, 20 minutes.
Per main course serving: 295 calories, 11 g total fat (3.5 g saturated fat), 15 mg cholesterol, 905 mg sodium, 3 g fiber.

Iodine

"When it rains, it pours," claims the Morton Salt motto. With the case of iodine, it's ironically true. Iodized salt is the most significant source of iodine in the United States—a nutrient once scarce in many parts of the country. Adding iodine to table salt began in 1924 in Michigan to help prevent the spread of goiter that was common in the Great Lakes region. The practice soon spread across the country.

RECOMMENDED INTAKE

RDA (Recommended Dietary Allowance)

Iodine (mcg/d)

Life-Stage	Children	Men	Women	Pregnancy	Lactation
1-3 years	90				
4-8 years	90				
9-13 years	120			220	290
14-18 years		150	150	220	290
19-30 years		150	150	220	290
31-50 years		150	150	220	290
51-70 years		150	150		
70+ years		150	150		

Source: The National Academy of Sciences

For optimal health consume 150 mcg per day.

WHAT IS IT?

The average adult body contains between 20 and 50 mg of iodine, most of it concentrated in the thyroid gland.

WHY YOU NEED IT

Hormones
Iodine helps your body form thyroid hormones, which are vital to physical growth and development. Thyroid hormones control metabolism, improve mental functioning and give you healthier hair, skin, nails and teeth.

MORE OR LESS?

Increased or decreased nutrient needs should always be discussed with your healthcare professional.

You may need higher than recommended amounts of iodine if you:
• *Take antithyroid medications, as these may prevent iodine from working properly.*
• *Live in an area that has low soil iodine (and rely on locally grown produce), restrict salt in your diet and don't eat a lot of fish.*

▶▶ Best natural food sources

■ Saltwater fish
■ Seafood

▶▶ Fortified foods

■ Iodized table salt

IF YOU GET TOO LITTLE

The average person only needs a teaspoon of iodine over the course of an entire lifetime. Deficiency of iodine is a world health problem but is relatively rare in industrialized countries with fortification programs. Severe iodine deficiency in the diet of a pregnant woman increases the risk of miscarriage and stillbirth; a baby who survives birth will likely suffer irreversible mental impairment. Mildly iodine-deficient children have learning disabilities and trouble concentrating. Iodine deficiency in adults leads to a variety of illnesses including hypothyroidism, goiter and cretinism.

IF YOU TAKE TOO MUCH

Excess iodine may cause acne, confusion, irregular heartbeat, goiter (swollen neck or throat) and bloody or tar-like stools. Less common symptoms include joint pain, swelling of the face and tongue and gum soreness. The minimum toxic dose is 2 mg.

(Continued...)

Did you know?

Food processors often use iodized salt and sanitizing solutions that contribute iodine indirectly to foods.

Worldwide distribution of iodine in the soil is extremely variable. Foods grown in the American Midwest, Southwest England, Europe, Russia, South America and parts of China have very low levels of iodine.

Supplement savvy

Only take iodine supplements if your healthcare provider has specifically prescribed them.

 Startling statistics

Iodine deficiency is the single most common cause of preventable mental retardation and brain damage in the world, affecting more than 50 million children.

KITCHEN CONNECTIONS

✔ *Iodine and anticaking agents added to salt can cause bitter flavors. Top chefs prefer sea salt when flavoring foods.*
✔ *Enjoy grilled cod or sea bass.*
✔ *Eggs and milk may be rich sources if iodine was added to the animal's feed.*

NUTRIENT THIEVES

▶ Poor soil is perhaps the only thief that robs iodine from foods.

SAUTEED SCALLOPS

Most seafood is rich in iodine, and scallops are no exception. The scallops you use here may be small, as in small bay scallops (about ½ inch in diameter) or larger, as in sea scallops (about 1½ to 2 inches in diameter). Either way, this is a delicious and simple way to prepare them.

3 tablespoons olive oil
1 lb. scallops
1 tablespoon butter
1 tablespoon chopped garlic
2 small shallots, chopped

❶ Heat olive oil in large skillet over medium-high heat until hot. Cook scallops quickly, stirring constantly about 3 to 5 minutes or until opaque. Transfer to warm platter.

❷ In large skillet, melt butter over medium heat. Sauté garlic and shallots 3 to 4 minutes or until golden. Pour sauce over scallops. Garnish with lemon slices and parsley. Serve immediately.

4 servings.
Preparation time: 10 minutes.
Ready to serve: 20 minutes.
Per serving: 250 calories, 14.5 g fat (3.5 g saturated fat), 45 mg cholesterol, 320 mg sodium, 0.5 g fiber.

Iron

Just as iron helps form the skeleton of a sky-scraper, it helps support your strength and vitality. For many people, especially women, it's hard to get enough iron. It's almost impossible for pregnant or breast-feeding women to meet their increased iron requirements. That's one of the rea-sons why prenatal supplements are so important. Before birth, a baby has just nine months to store up enough iron to last until it's time to start solid foods. Breast milk is naturally low in iron. New moms also need to replace iron stores that were depleted during pregnancy and to make up for the

RECOMMENDED INTAKE

RDA (Recommended Dietary Allowance)

Iron (mg/d)

Life-Stage	Children	Men	Women	Pregnancy	Lactation
1-3 years	7				
4-8 years	10				
9-13 years	8			27	10
14-18 years		11	15	27	10
19-30 years		8	18	27	9
31-50 years		8	18	27	9
51-70 years		8	8		
70+ years		8	8		

Source: The National Academy of Sciences

**For optimal health consume 10 to 30 mg per day.
Children, men and postmenopausal women require lower levels of iron.**

additional blood lost during delivery and recovery from the birthing process. Women with heavy menstrual blood losses may need the same high levels of iron (30 mg/day) as pregnant women.

WHAT IT IS

Iron is the most abundant element on earth, yet is needed in only minute amounts for humans. Iron is found in both animal and plant foods. Animal foods contain heme sources of iron and plant foods have nonheme iron. About 20 to 30 percent of the heme iron is absorbed, compared to only 2 to 5 percent of nonheme iron. Iron must be in ferrous form to be absorbed; it's the hydrochloric acid in your stomach that processes this conversion.

WHY YOU NEED IT

Metabolism
How much iron you have determines how much oxygen gets to the rest of your body tissues.

Hormones
Thyroid hormones require iron for production.

Immune System
Iron is critical in building and maintaining a healthy immune system.

MORE OR LESS?

Increased or decreased nutrient needs should always be discussed with your healthcare professional.

You may need higher than recommended amounts of iron if you have:
* *heavy menstrual periods*
* *medical conditions that cause blood loss (wounds, surgery, bleeding ulcers)*
* *a strict vegan diet*
* *cholesterol-lowering medication for long-term use*

You may need less than recommended amounts of iron if you have:
* *Hemochromatosis—a genetic abnormality that causes a higher than normal absorption of iron*

▶▶ **Best natural food sources**

- Beef
- Bran
- Clams
- Oysters
- Soybeans (cooked)
- Spinach (cooked)

▶▶ **Fortified foods**

- Bread
- Farina
- Oatmeal
- Pasta
- Some ready-to-eat cereals
- White rice

(Continued...)

IF YOU GET TOO LITTLE

Iron deficiency (anemia) is probably the most common nutritional deficiency in the United States. Symptoms of anemia include fatigue, inability to concentrate, pale skin tone, cracks in the corners of the mouth, eye inflammation, mouth ulcers, hair loss and thin or brittle fingernails. Pregnant women with iron deficiency are more prone to infection after delivery, premature delivery and low birthweight babies.

IF YOU TAKE TOO MUCH

Too much iron may cause constipation, upset stomach, abdominal pain or bloody diarrhea. Long-term high intakes may lead to deterioration of the stomach lining and liver damage. Minimum toxic dose is 30 mg. In children, a toxic dose of just 3 g (the amount in 10 prenatal vitamins) can be severe enough to cause convulsions, coma or death. Early signs of iron overdose may not appear for up to 60 minutes or more. Do not delay going to the emergency room while waiting for signs to appear.

(!) Think twice!

Too much iron is as damaging as too little. Excess iron causes oxidation and free radical damage that has been linked to heart disease and some cancers. Take supplements only when recommended by your healthcare provider.

(?) Did you know?

Tea (iced or hot) is so effective at blocking iron absorption that it is sometimes used by people with excess iron buildup.

The average American diet provides about 6 mg of iron per 1,000 calories. That means you need to eat at least 2,500 calories a day to get enough iron—or be especially vigilant about choosing iron-rich foods.

Stools commonly become dark green or black when iron preparations are taken by mouth. This is caused by unabsorbed iron and is harmless. However, in rare cases, black stools of a sticky consistency may occur along with other side effects such as red streaks in the stool, cramping, soreness or sharp pains in the stomach or abdominal area. Check with your healthcare professional immediately if these side effects appear.

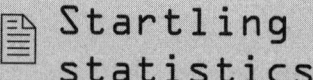

Startling statistics

In children, a toxic dose of just 3 g (the amount in 10 prenatal vitamins) can be severe enough to cause convulsions, coma or death.

KITCHEN CONNECTIONS

✔ *Cast-iron pots and pans add a small but significant amount of iron to the foods cooked in them.*

✔ *Combine a food high in vitamin C with a plant food that contains iron to dramatically increase absorption. For example, add some orange sections to a spinach salad or mix red or green peppers into your favorite bean dish.*

✔ *Stock your pantry with canned kidney and pinto beans. Rinse and toss into salads, dips or tortillas for extra iron.*

NUTRIENT THIEVES

▶ Low stomach acid or taking antacids will diminish iron absorption. Phosphates (found in meats and soft drinks), oxalates (found in spinach, chard and other vegetables), and phytates (found in whole grains), all can bind iron complexes or salts that will not otherwise be absorbed. Soy protein is being researched, as it may also reduce iron absorption.

Supplement savvy

Don't take any iron-containing supplement with a glass of tea or coffee. The tannins in these beverages—especially tea—grab onto the iron and block its absorption.

Liquid forms of iron supplements tend to stain the teeth. To prevent this reaction, mix each dose in water or fruit juice and drink through a straw to help keep the iron supplement from getting on your teeth.

Do not take iron supplements and antacids or calcium supplements at the same time. It is best to space doses of these products 1 to 2 hours apart to get the full benefit from each medicine or dietary supplement.

Magnesium

A special region in Greece, called Magnesia, was frequently visited in ancient times because of the magical powers within a salty, white powder. Ever heard of "Milk of Magnesia"? Magnesium works as an antacid in small doses and as a laxative in large amounts. This multi-purpose mineral is also what early photographers used to create light flashes before the days of flashcubes or electronic flashes.

RECOMMENDED INTAKE

RDA (Recommended Dietary Allowance)

Magnesium (mg/d)

Life-Stage	Children	Men	Women	Pregnancy	Lactation
1-3 years	80				
4-8 years	130				
9-13 years	240			400	360
14-18 years		410	360	400	360
19-30 years		400	310	350	310
31-50 years		420	320	360	320
51-70 years		420	320		
70+ years		420	320		

Source: The National Academy of Sciences

For optimal health consume 300 to 500 mg per day.

What Is It?

Magnesium is the trigger that activates more than 300 enzymes. Enzymes regulate many body functions, including energy production and muscle contractions. Magnesium works as a signal for muscles to contract and relax. And when the muscles that line major blood vessels contract, it impacts your blood pressure. Magnesium helps just about every other chemical in your body do its job. Magnesium is mainly an intracellular (inside the cells) ion. Most magnesium in the body is in the skeleton, 20 to 30 percent is in muscle, and only about 2 percent is outside of cells.

Why You Need It

Bones & Teeth
In conjunction with calcium, magnesium helps build strong bones and teeth.

Circulatory System
In the heart tissue, magnesium functions as a calcium channel-blocker, preventing the influx of too much calcium into the cells. Magnesium also helps regulate body temperature.

Metabolism
Magnesium regulates cellular ion balance, keeping potassium in and sodium out of the cells. It also regulates cellular glucose metabolism, protein digestion and certain hormone receptor signal transmissions.

More or Less?

Increased or decreased nutrient needs should always be discussed with your healthcare professional.

You may need higher than recommended amounts of magnesium if you are:
* *Alcoholic*
* *Type 2 diabetic*
* *Taking diuretic medications*

You may need less than recommended amounts of magnesium if you have:
* *Kidney disease (Magnesium supplements are not recommended; check with your doctor for medications that prevent magnesium deficiency.)*

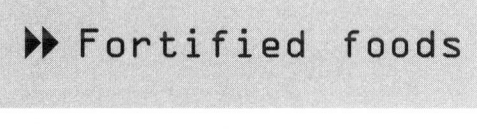

▶▶ Best natural food sources

No food provides 25 percent or more of the RDA in one serving.

Foods that provide 10 to 24 percent of the RDA include:

- Broccoli
- Dry beans
- Dry peas
- Halibut
- Lentils
- Nonfat yogurt
- Nut butters
- Nuts
- Pumpkin seeds
- Skin-on potatoes
- Spinach
- Whole grains

▶▶ Fortified foods

- None

(Continued...)

IF YOU GET TOO LITTLE

Marginal intakes of magnesium over time can lead to an increased risk for many chronic diseases including heart disease, high blood pressure, diabetes, osteoporosis, asthma, migraine headaches, PMS and kidney stones. Common symptoms of deficiency include irritability, personality changes, loss of appetite, weakness, hair loss and swollen gums.

IF YOU TAKE TOO MUCH

Too much supplemental magnesium may cause nausea, flushed skin, fatigue, vomiting, low blood pressure, muscle weakness and irregular heartbeat.

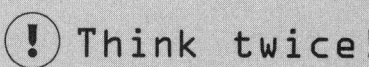
Think twice!

Drinking water is an important source of magnesium, especially in hard water areas. Your body absorbs magnesium better from water than from foods.

Did you know?

Since the 1960s, researchers have known that people who live in areas where the water is "hard" often have lower rates of heart disease and stroke. ("Hard" water contains more calcium, magnesium and other minerals than "soft" water.)

KITCHEN CONNECTIONS

✔ *Use a variety of beans in soups.*
✔ *Add a sprinkle of nuts to oatmeal.*
✔ *Have a grilled halibut sandwich on a whole-wheat hoagie roll.*

NUTRIENT THIEVES

▶ Meals high in protein or fat, a diet high in phosphorus or calcium (calcium and magnesium can compete) or alcohol use may decrease magnesium absorption.

Supplement savvy

Magnesium supplements are not needed by most people. If you do require a supplement, avoid "enteric-coated" tablets that are not absorbed well.

OVEN-ROASTED SPUDS

Keep the skin on your potatoes to keep the magnesium with them. Try an oil infused with an herb, such as garlic or rosemary, to enhance these crusty, quick-cooked potatoes.

10 to 12 medium new red potatoes,
    cut into 1-inch pieces
1 tablespoon salt
¼ cup olive oil
2 tablespoons chopped fresh rosemary
    or 2 teaspoons dried
1 tablespoon chopped fresh dill
    or 1 teaspoon dried
⅛ teaspoon kosher (coarse) salt
⅛ teaspoon freshly ground pepper

❶ Heat oven to 400°F. Spray 15x10x1-inch baking sheet with nonstick cooking spray.

❷ In large pot, cover potatoes with water; add salt. Bring to a boil over high heat. Reduce heat to medium; boil 10 minutes or until tender.

❸ Pour in olive oil, rosemary and dill. Season with salt and pepper. Toss gently to coat potatoes. Spread on baking sheet. Bake 5 minutes. Reduce heat to 375°F. Turn potatoes with spatula. Bake an additional 15 minutes or until potatoes are nicely browned and cooked through.

4 to 6 servings.

Preparation time: 20 minutes.

Ready to serve: 45 minutes.

Per serving: 355 calories, 14 g fat (2 g saturated fat), 0 mg cholesterol, 600 mg sodium, 5 g fiber.

Manganese

Manganese isn't a glamorous nutrient, but it is shrouded in magical mystery. Actually, the word manganese comes from the Greek word for magic. We don't know much about manganese yet, because few scientists are interested in studying it. The first reported deficiency of manganese was not noted until 1972.

More people are adopting a vegetarian lifestyle, and there is some concern that vegetarians' bodies are storing too much manganese over time. This happens because vegetarians have naturally higher intakes of manganese with their plant-based diets.

RECOMMENDED INTAKE

AI (Adequate Intake)

Manganese (mg/d)

Life-Stage	Children	Men	Women	Pregnancy	Lactation
1-3 years	1.2				
4-8 years	1.5				
9-13 years		1.9	1.6	2.0	2.6
14-18 years		2.2	1.6	2.0	2.6
19-30 years		2.3	1.8	2.0	2.6
31-50 years		2.3	1.8	2.0	2.6
51-70 years		2.3	1.8		
70+ years		2.3	1.8		

Source: The National Academy of Sciences

For optimal health consume 2.5 to 5 mg per day.

Vegetarians are also more likely to develop iron deficiency anemia, which tends to increase the amount of manganese that is absorbed. Until more research tests this theory, it might be best for vegetarians to avoid supplements with high levels of manganese.

WHAT IS IT?

Like copper, molybdenum and other minerals, manganese is an essential part of many enzymes. This mineral is present in a wide variety of foods.

WHY YOU NEED IT

Bones & Teeth
Manganese helps in the development of bones, teeth and joints.

Hormones
Female sex hormones and thyroid hormones are dependent on manganese to work properly.

MORE OR LESS?

Increased or decreased nutrient needs should always be discussed with your healthcare professional.

You may need higher than recommended amounts of manganese if you:
* *Eat mostly refined and highly processed foods*

You might need less manganese if you are:
* *Vegetarian*

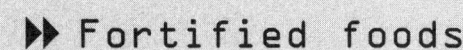

▶▶ Best natural food sources

- Kale
- Lentils
- Pineapple
- Strawberries
- Tea
- Whole grains

▶▶ Fortified foods

- None

IF YOU GET TOO LITTLE

The first report of manganese deficiency was noted in 1972 and is extremely rare. Symptoms may include dizziness, skin problems and slowed growth of hair and nails.

IF YOU TAKE TOO MUCH

Large doses may cause depression, delusions, hallucinations, impotence and insomnia. There is known minimum toxic dose.

(Continued...)

! Think twice!

Large amounts of manganese may interfere with iron absorption.

Supplement savvy

Supplements of manganese, other than amounts found in a multivitamin/mineral supplement are not recommended.

? Did you know?

One form of the antioxidant enzyme, super-oxide dimutase, contains manganese. Levels of this enzyme are high in alcoholics and may help to protect the liver from damage by alcohol.

KITCHEN CONNECTIONS

✔ *Top a salad with sliced strawberries and pineapple.*
✔ *Make time for tea with whole-wheat finger sandwiches.*

NUTRIENT THIEVES

▶ Large amounts of calcium and/or phosphorus will interfere with manganese absorption. Heavy milk drinkers or consumers of soft drinks may need additional manganese.

SPRING FRUIT CRISP

If you feel adventurous, try some other fruits in this great crisp. But to start, the rhubarb and strawberries are wonderful, and the strawberries are a natural source of manganese.

CRISP
2 cups diced rhubarb
2 cups strawberries, hulled
1 cup sugar
2 tablespoons all-purpose flour
⅛ teaspoon ground cloves

TOPPING
1 cup packed brown sugar
¾ cup all-purpose flour
½ teaspoon cinnamon
Dash ground cloves
6 tablespoons butter, chilled
½ cup chopped pecans

1. Heat oven to 350°F. Spray 9-inch square pan with nonstick cooking spray.
2. In large bowl, toss rhubarb and strawberries with sugar, flour and cloves. Pour into pan. Set aside.
3. In small bowl, mix brown sugar, flour, cinnamon and cloves. Cut in butter with pastry blender or fingers until mixture crumbles. Stir in pecans.
4. Spread nut mixture over rhubarb and strawberries.
5. Bake 45 minutes or until golden brown and bubbly.

8 servings
Preparation time: 20 minutes.
Ready to serve: 1 hour, 5 minutes.
Per serving: 390 calories, 14 g fat (6 g saturated fat), 25 mg cholesterol, 70 mg sodium, 2.5 g fiber.

Molybdenum

olybdenum is the least known of all essential minerals. It's also one of the scarcest elements in the earth's crust. Like other minerals, the molybdenum content of the soil affects the amount of the mineral found in food. Molybdcnum is also found in most water. Most public water supplies are estimated to contribute between 2 and 8 mcg of molybdenum daily.

WHAT IS IT?

Molybdenum is an essential trace mineral. It is needed for the proper function of certain enzyme-dependent processes.

RECOMMENDED INTAKE

RDA (Recommended Dietary Allowance)

Molybdenum (mcg/d)

Life-Stage	Children	Men	Women	Pregnancy	Lactation
1-3 years	17				
4-8 years	22				
9-13 years	34			50	50
14-18 years		43	43	50	50
19-30 years		45	45	50	50
31-50 years		45	45	50	50
51-70 years		45	45		
70+ years		45	45		

Source: The National Academy of Sciences

For optimal health consume 75 to 250 mcg per day.

WHY YOU NEED IT

The main function of molybdenum is to help make enzymes that perform a variety of functions. Two of the most important roles of these molybdenum-containing enzymes are to help your body use stored iron and be able to burn fat for energy.

MORE OR LESS?

Increased or decreased nutrient needs should always be discussed with your healthcare professional.

You may need higher than recommended amounts of molybdenum if you have:
* *Wilson's disease (molybdenum is sometimes used to treat copper toxicity)*

▶▶ Best natural food sources

- Dark leafy green vegetables
- Legumes
- Milk

▶▶ Fortified foods

- Cold cereals
- Enriched breads

IF YOU GET TOO LITTLE

Molybdenum deficiency is extremely rare and has only been reported in people on long-term tube or IV feedings. Symptoms include rapid heartbeat, headache, night blindness, nausea and vomiting.

IF YOU TAKE TOO MUCH

Too much molybdenum may cause excessive loss of copper in urine. Minimum toxic dose is 10 mg.

(?) Did you know?

Molybdenum is part of an enzyme that helps detoxify sulfites found naturally in protein foods and used as a preservative in some foods and drugs. Some people are sensitive to sulfites, but extra molybdenum does not help eliminate or reduce this sensitivity, so supplements are of no use.

KITCHEN CONNECTIONS

- ✔ *Mix granola with buckwheat, oats and wheat germ.*
- ✔ *Add garbanzo beans to a leafy green salad.*

NUTRIENT THIEVES

▶ Refined foods and overused soil decrease the amount of molybdenum in foods.

 ### Supplement savvy

Molybdenum supplements are not recommended.

Phosphorus

Do you consume soft drinks or take antacids that contain aluminum hydroxide? Check the ingredient list. If you find it listed on the label, you might be disrupting your body's delicate calcium/phosphorus balance. Too much aluminum hydroxide may decrease your absorption of phosphorus, which can lead to weakened bones. Processed foods are another culprit, frequently adding phosphorus-containing preservatives to your diet. Milk provides the best ratio of phosphorus to calcium.

RECOMMENDED INTAKE

RDA (Recommended Dietary Allowance)

Phosphorus (mg/d)

Life-Stage	Children	Men	Women	Pregnancy	Lactation
1-3 years	460				
4-8 years	500				
9-13 years	1250			1250	1250
14-18 years		1250	1250	1250	1250
19-30 years		700	700	700	700
31-50 years		700	700	700	700
51-70 years		700	700		
70+ years		700	700		

Source: The National Academy of Sciences

For optimal health aim for 800 to 1,200 mg per day.

What Is It?

Phosphorus is second only to its mineral relative, calcium, in abundance in the body. In the form of phosphates, it is a major component of the mineral phase of bone and is involved in almost all metabolic processes. It also plays an important role in cell metabolism. Inhalation of phosphorus vapor by workers in chemical industries may cause decay of the mandible bone of the jaw.

Why You Need It

Bones & Teeth
Phosphorus helps build strong bones and teeth.

Metabolism
Phosphorus helps release energy from protein, fat and carbohydrate during the digestion of food. It also forms genetic material, cell membranes and many enzymes.

More or Less?

Increased or decreased nutrient needs should always be discussed with your healthcare professional.

You may need higher than recommended amounts of phosphorus if you are:
* Age 70 or older
* On a severely limited or restricted diet
* Taking large amounts of aluminum-containing antacids

▶▶ Best natural food sources

- ■ Carp
- ■ Chocolate milk
- ■ Low-fat or nonfat yogurt
- ■ Mackerel
- ■ Salmon (canned)
- ■ Swordfish

▶▶ Fortified foods

- ■ None

If You Get Too Little

A diet deficient in phosphorus is extremely rare. Signs of deficiency can include weakness, loss of appetite, bone pain, joint stiffness, numbness, confusion and speech problems.

If You Take Too Much

Too much phosphorus may cause side effects including shortness of breath, irregular heartbeat and seizures. The minimum toxic dose of phosphorus is thought to be 12,000 mg.

(Continued...)

! Think twice!

Antacids that contain large amounts of aluminum can block phosphorus absorption.

? Did you know?

Most people get phosphorus in the form of food additives such as monocalcium phosphate and sodium aluminum phosphate. One diet soft drink has about 30 mg of phosphorus.

📄 Startling statistics

The average American consumes 7 to 10 times the adult requirement for phosphorus daily.

KITCHEN CONNECTIONS

✔ *Use low-fat chocolate milk when making pudding.*
✔ *Enjoy a turkey and cheddar sandwich on whole-grain bread.*

NUTRIENT THIEVES

▶ Caffeine causes increased phosphorus excretion by your kidneys.

Supplement savvy

Phosphorus supplements are not recommended.

SWORDFISH SOUVLAKI

Oregano-laced souvlaki is a Greek marinade usually used with lamb, but souvlaki used with sword-fish is popular too, and the fish is a good source of phosphorus. Bay leaves dress up the skewers and contribute a subtle fragrance.

20 to 24 fresh or dried bay leaves
3 tablespoons fresh lemon juice
3 tablespoons dry white wine
1 tablespoon extra-virgin olive oil
1½ tablespoons chopped fresh oregano or
    1½ teaspoons dried
1 garlic clove, minced
½ teaspoon salt
⅛ teaspoon freshly ground pepper
1¼-lb. swordfish steak (1¼ inches thick),
    skin removed, cut into 1¼-inch chunks
Lemon wedges

❶ If using dried bay leaves, soak in water 30 minutes.

❷ In small bowl, whisk lemon juice, wine, oil, oregano, garlic, salt and pepper. Reserve 3 tablespoons of this mixture for basting. Place swordfish in shallow glass dish. Add remaining marinade; turn to coat. Refrigerate, covered, 20 to 30 minutes, turning occasionally.

❸ Heat grill. Thread swordfish onto 4 (10- or 12-inch) skewers, placing one bay leaf between each piece of swordfish.

❹ Lightly oil grill rack. Place skewers on gas grill over medium-high heat or charcoal grill over medium-hot coals. Cover grill and cook, turning occasionally and basting with reserved marinade, 8 to 12 minutes or until swordfish is opaque in center. Garnish with lemon wedges.

4 servings.
Preparation time: 20 minutes.
Ready to serve: 40 minutes.
Per serving: 185 calories, 8 g total fat (2 g saturated fat), 75 mg cholesterol, 215 mg sodium, 0 g fiber.

Potassium

Believe it or not, bananas are not nature's best source of potassium. Although a balanced diet usually supplies all the potassium a person needs, potassium supplements seem popular because illness or treatment with certain medicines can dramatically deplete potassium stores in your body.

WHAT IS IT?

The silvery white metal is so soft it can be cut with a regular kitchen knife. Potassium is found in nature in large quantities. It is the eighth most abundant element in the crust of the earth. In fact, potassium is part of all plant and animal tissue as well as a vital ingredient in fertile soil.

WHY YOU NEED IT

Metabolism
Potassium also affects blood pressure by relaxing the artery walls. Relaxed walls allow blood to flow smoothly, which helps keep your blood pressure low. Your body contains about 5 ounces of potassium.

RECOMMENDED INTAKE

There is no RDA or AI developed yet for potassium. The estimated minimum requirement for healthy adults is 2,000 mg per day according to the recommendations of the National Academy of Sciences. However, there is considerable evidence that potassium from foods has a beneficial effect in reducing hypertension. Eating lots of fruits and vegetables, as is frequently recommended, would raise the optimal potassium intake to 3,500 mg per day.

For optimal health consume 2,000 to 5,000 mg per day.

MORE OR LESS?

Increased or decreased nutrient needs should always be discussed with your healthcare professional.

You may need higher than recommended amounts of potassium if you are:
- *Fasting*
- *Taking certain diuretic medications—check with your health care provider*

►► Best natural food sources

- 100% bran cereal
- Apricots (dried)
- Avocados
- Bananas
- Black beans
- Carp
- Catfish
- Chard
- Cod
- Dry peas (cooked)
- Flounder
- Kidney beans
- Lentils
- Lima beans
- Milk
- Mullet
- Orange juice
- Peaches (dried)
- Plantains
- Pomegranate
- Pork
- Potatoes
- Prune juice
- Prunes
- Pumpkin
- Soybeans
- Spinach
- Squash
- Tomato juice
- Tomatoes (cooked)
- Veal
- Yogurt

►► Fortified foods

- None

IF YOU GET TOO LITTLE

There are dozens of symptoms of potassium deficiency ranging from fatigue, muscle cramping, weakness, bloating, loss of appetite, drowsiness, numbness and tingling and increased thirst to heartbeat irregularities and eventually coma or death. Chronic potassium deficiency is thought to play a significant role in increasing the risk of high blood pressure.

IF YOU TAKE TOO MUCH

A healthy person can't get a toxic amount of potassium from foods. People with advanced kidney disease, adrenal hormone dysfunction or major infections or those suffering shock after an injury can have too much potassium leak out of their cells and into the blood at abnormally high levels. Symptoms of potassium overload include nausea, vomiting, diarrhea and abdominal cramps. Large amounts from supplements may cause increased heart rate, low blood pressure, convulsions, paralysis of limbs and cardiac arrest.

(Continued...)

(!) Think twice!

Potassium supplements may increase the risk of hyperkalemia (high blood levels of potassium), which may worsen or cause heart problems.

(?) Did you know?

Many salt substitutes use potassium as a replacement for sodium. If you have heart disease or decreased kidney function you should never use salt substitutes without the specific advice of your healthcare provider.

Startling statistics

The sudden death that can occur when you fast or starve is often the result of heart failure caused by too little potassium.

KITCHEN CONNECTIONS

✔ *Add sliced bananas to bran cereal*
✔ *Make chili with extra tomatoes and kidney beans*

NUTRIENT THIEVES

▶ Potassium is easily lost in the cooking and processing of foods.

Supplement savvy

Supplements of potassium are not recommended unless specifically prescribed by your healthcare provider.

BLACK BEAN, CORN & GREEN CHILE QUESADILLAS

So many food sources offer potassium, it's easy to get enough in your diet. These quesadillas, with their black beans, make the task fun.

2 medium ears corn
2 Anaheim or New Mexico chiles
1 (15-oz.) can black beans, rinsed, drained
¼ cup thinly sliced green onions
1 red jalapeño pepper, seeded, minced
1 tablespoon lime juice
½ teaspoon salt
4 (10-inch) flour tortillas
2 cups (8 oz.) shredded Monterey Jack cheese

1 Remove silk from corn, leaving husks intact. Place corn and chiles on gas grill over medium-high heat or on charcoal grill 4 to 6 inches from medium-high coals. Grill chiles 8 to 10 minutes, turning when first side is charred. Grill corn about 12 minutes, turning ¼ turn every 3 minutes.

2 Remove chiles from heat; place in paper bag 5 minutes to loosen blackened skin. Remove corn from heat; let cool. Husk; remove kernels from cob. Place in medium bowl. Scrape skin from chiles; remove seeds and inner membranes. Chop chiles and place in bowl.

3 Add black beans, onions, jalapeño, lime juice and salt. Divide mixture evenly among tortillas; spread on one half of each tortilla. Sprinkle each filled half with ½ cup of the cheese. Fold tortilla over filling.

4 Heat large skillet or griddle (make sure handle is heat-resistant) on gas grill over medium-high heat or on charcoal grill 4 to 6 inches from medium-high coals, or on stove over medium-high heat. Cook each tortilla 4 minutes per side or until browned, turning once. Cut into quarters; serve with salsa, if desired.

8 servings.
Preparation time: 15 minutes.
Ready to serve: 47 minutes.
Per serving: 290 calories, 11.5 g total fat (6 g saturated fat), 25 mg cholesterol, 570 mg sodium, 4.5 g fiber.

Selenium

Your body's most abundant natural antioxidant is an enzyme that is dependent on selenium. Selenium has been identified as an essential nutrient for only 30 years. Lots of research is in the works, looking at the role this mineral may play in reducing your risk of several major diseases including cancer, heart disease, kidney disease and male infertility.

You can't accurately estimate the amount of selenium you get from foods since the same foods can vary widely in their selenium content. The best way to measure your selenium intake is through a blood

RECOMMENDED INTAKE

RDA (Recommended Dietary Allowance)
Selenium (mcg/d)

Life-Stage	Children	Men	Women	Pregnancy	Lactation
1-3 years	20				
4-8 years	30				
9-13 years	40			60	70
14-18 years		55	55	60	70
19-30 years		55	55	60	70
31-50 years		55	55	60	70
51-70 years		55	55		
70+ years		55	55		

Source: The National Academy of Sciences

For optimal health consume 200 mcg per day.

test and analysis of toenail clippings. If your selenium intake is low, less of this mineral will be deposited into your nails.

WHAT IS IT?

Selenium is a trace element found to a varying extent in soil. It enters the human diet through plants such as corn and through the meat of animals grazing on vegetation containing selenium. Products from selenium-rich soils of the United States' plains and mountain regions carry proportionately more selenium than those coming from the Upper Midwest, Northeast and Florida, where selenium soil concentration is low.

WHY YOU NEED IT

Antioxidant Actions
Selenium is a powerful antioxidant that protects red blood cells and cell membranes from free radical damage. It also works with and helps vitamin E with other antioxidant functions. It may help protect against some of the damaging effects of ultraviolet light.

Hormones
Selenium is needed to activate thyroid hormones.

Immune System
Selenium is also essential for healthy immune functioning. As a result, selenium supplementation has reduced the incidence of hepatitis in deficient populations. In elderly people, selenium has been found to stimulate the activity of white blood cells—primary components of the immune system.

MORE OR LESS?

Increased or decreased nutrient needs should always be discussed with your healthcare professional.

You may need higher than recommended amounts of selenium if you have:

* *Keshan's disease—a heart muscle disease that affects people who grow all their own foods in areas of low selenium.*

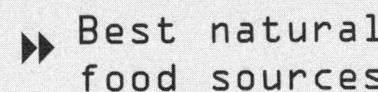

▶▶ **Best natural food sources**

Accurate levels of selenium in cultivated plant foods are not available as selenium content varies with the soil levels of this mineral.

■ Haddock
■ Salmon

▶▶ **Fortified foods**

■ None

(Continued...)

IF YOU GET TOO LITTLE

While most people probably don't take in enough selenium, deficiencies are rare. Soils in some areas are selenium-deficient and people who eat foods grown primarily on selenium-poor soils are at risk for deficiency.

IF YOU TAKE TOO MUCH

Too much supplemental selenium can cause hair loss, fingernail loss, fatigue, nausea and nerve damage. Minimum toxic dose is 700 micrograms.

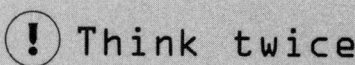 Think twice!

Most experts agree that more research is needed before recommending selenium supplements.

(?) Did you know?

High-selenium yeast supplements sold in health food stores are made by spraying yeast with inorganic sodium selenite. This form of selenium is not very well absorbed.

KITCHEN CONNECTIONS

✔ *Grill salmon with seasoned wheat germ breading.*
✔ *Enjoy a gyro made with shaved lamb and whole-wheat pita bread.*

NUTRIENT THIEVES

▸ Most selenium in foods (for example, white rice and white flour) is lost during processing.

 Supplement savvy

Supplementation with separate selenium tablets is not recommended. The amount of selenium found in most vitamin/mineral supplements is plenty.

POACHED SALMON STEAKS

Salmon is filled with nutrients, of which the mineral selenium is one. Here's how to poach salmon—a healthy way to cook it. Use a large skillet with a lid for poaching thick fish steaks. Add one of the suggested sauces or one of your own.

4 (8-oz.) salmon steaks, about 1 inch thick
Boiling water
2 tablespoons fresh lemon juice
2 bay leaves

❶ Spray large skillet with nonstick cooking spray. Arrange steaks in skillet in one layer.

❷ Pour enough boiling water over fish to come halfway up sides of steaks. Pour lemon juice over fish; tuck bay leaves under fish.

❸ Bring to a simmer over medium heat. Cover and cook 8 to 10 minutes or until fish flakes easily with fork.

❹ Use wide, slotted spatula to remove fish from skillet. Drain on paper towels. Discard bay leaves.

❺ Serve hot or chilled garnished with lemon wedges, Dilled Mayonnaise or Speedy Provencale, if desired.

4 servings.
Preparation time: 5 minutes.
Ready to serve: 15 minutes.
Per serving: 170 calories, 7 g fat (2 g saturated fat), 80 mg cholesterol, 70 mg sodium, 0 g fiber.

Dilled Mayonnaise Sauce
In large bowl, combine ¾ cup mayonnaise with ¼ cup plain yogurt and 2 tablespoons fresh dill. Season with ground white pepper. Store covered in refrigerator.

Provencale Sauce
Stir 2 tablespoons chopped roasted red bell peppers and 2 tablespoons chopped niçoise olives into 1 cup drained chopped Italian-style tomatoes. Store covered in refrigerator.

Sodium

Many of us reach for the salt shaker as soon as our plate is served. You don't need that extra sodium, but will it harm you? The answer to that question is still being debated.

Sodium is the nutrient most frequently associated as a villain in blood pressure. Current research shows some individuals have much greater blood pressure responses to salt than others. About half those individuals who have high blood pressure are "salt sensitive." But only 10 percent of the total American population falls into this category. Since there is no harm in moderately cutting back on dietary sodium, reduction is widely recommended.

There's also a theory that high levels of sodium over time may cause rising blood pressure as you age. So if your blood pressure is normal now, cutting back to a reasonable amount of sodium may help keep it that way.

WHAT IS IT?

Sodium is the main positively charged ion in your blood and other body fluids. About one-third of the sodium in your body is enmeshed in the mineralized crystals found in your bones and teeth. If you ate only unprocessed foods and added no table salt, you'd still get enough sodium to meet normal needs. Just 400 to 500 milligrams of sodium per day is enough to keep your body fluids and blood pressure in balance. Of course, if you are extremely active, have a fever, prolonged diarrhea or vomiting, you need extra sodium. That's why soup, broth and saltine crackers are frequently recommended during illness.

WHY YOU NEED IT

Cardiovascular System
The best-known function of sodium is to help regulate blood pressure. It also aids in muscle contraction.

Fluid Balance
Sodium, along with potassium and chloride, help regulate fluid balance and keep your blood pH normal.

Nervous System & Brain
The electrical current that helps send nerve impulses through your body is stimulated by the positive charge of sodium molecules.

RECOMMENDED INTAKE

Figuring out what a "reasonable" amount of sodium is has turned out to be a major public health debate. Many public and private organizations including the U.S. Department of Agriculture and the American Heart Association say Americans should consume no more than 2,400 mg of sodium a day. A more reasonable estimate of moderate sodium for healthy adults with normal blood pressure is probably in the range of 4,000 to 5,000 mg per day.

More or Less?

Increased or decreased nutrient needs should always be discussed with your healthcare professional.

You may need higher than recommended amounts of sodium if you have:

* *Heavy, prolonged sweating*
* *Chronic or severe diarrhea*

You may need less than recommended amounts of sodium if you have:

* *Kidney disease*
* *Salt-sensitive high blood pressure*

If You Get Too Little

Sodium deficiency is extremely rare. Prolonged heavy sweating, chronic diarrhea or extended use of diuretics may lead to sodium depletion. Symptoms include a sudden drop in blood pressure and shock.

If You Take Too Much

There is no established minimum toxic dose of sodium since excess levels vary by individual and health status. Too much sodium may cause fluid retention, swelling, and high blood pressure in people who are sodium-sensitive.

▶▶ Best natural food sources

■ None, though all foods contain some sodium

▶▶ Fortified foods

■ Most processed foods have moderate to high amounts of added sodium

(!) Think twice!

Many over-the-counter medications are full of sodium. If you are on a strict sodium restriction, be sure to read and check all food, supplement and medication labels for sodium content.

Never use salt substitutes without your doctor's permission if you are on medication to lower high blood pressure. Many salt substitutes contain large amounts of potassium, which may be dangerous to some individuals.

(Continued...)

? Did you know?

It's hard to eat less than 5,000 milligrams of sodium if you rely on processed convenience foods and/or often eat meals away from home.

Salt is an acquired taste. The more you eat, the more you want. It can take up to six weeks for you to gradually lose your desire for salty foods.

🝡 Supplement savvy

Sports beverages provide modest levels of sodium and other electrolytes that are needed by individuals with a high sweat rate or those exercising in very hot and humid conditions. Salt tablets are never recommended; they are too concentrated and do not provide the fluid base that is most important in rehydration.

📄 Startling statistics

The average American consumes between 2 and 4 teaspoons of salt per day. Of course, most of that is what's added during food processing and not what is sprinkled on at mealtime.

KITCHEN CONNECTIONS

✔ *If you need to add salt, do it at the table, not during cooking. Salt added to foods after cooking provides a huge amount of flavor, because the salt is placed right on your taste buds when it goes into your mouth. Salt or sodium-based seasonings that are cooked into food or added as preservatives don't have the same dramatic effect.*

✔ *Choose reduced sodium condensed soups and broths for making casseroles.*

✔ *Experiment with spice blends and herbs to add flavor and zest to food.*

✔ *Go easy on high-sodium condiments such as ketchup, chili sauce and relishes.*

HERB GARDEN SALAD

Most people want less sodium rather than more. Here's a way to get less in your salad dressing, and still enjoy great flavor. Plus, herbs give the salad greens a delightful herbal fragrance. To showcase the flavor of the herbs, use a delicate lettuce like Boston, rather than stronger-tasting salad greens like dandelion and radicchio.

VINAIGRETTE
4 teaspoons tarragon vinegar or white wine vinegar
2 tablespoons finely chopped shallots
½ teaspoon Dijon mustard
¼ teaspoon salt
⅛ teaspoon freshly ground pepper
Dash of sugar
¼ cup extra-virgin olive oil

SALAD
1 garlic clove, halved
2 medium heads butterhead (Boston or Bibb)
  lettuce leaves, torn into bite-sized pieces (8 cups)
1 cup fresh Italian parsley leaves, torn into
  ½-inch pieces
1 cup assorted herb leaves, torn into
  ½-inch pieces (burnet, chervil, lovage, tarragon, etc.)
½ cup chopped chives
12 unsprayed edible flowers
  (chive blossoms, nasturtiums, etc.), if desired

❶ In small jar with tight-fitting lid, combine vinegar, shallots, mustard, salt, pepper and sugar. Cover jar; shake to blend. Add oil; shake to blend. (Dressing can be prepared up to 2 days ahead. Cover and refrigerate.)

❷ Rub large salad bowl with cut sides of garlic clove. Place lettuce, parsley, assorted herbs and chives in bowl. Just before serving, drizzle dressing over salad; toss well. Garnish with flowers.

6 (2-cup) servings.
Preparation time: 25 minutes.
Ready to serve: 25 minutes.
Per serving: 95 calories, 9.5 g total fat (1.5 g saturated fat), 0 mg cholesterol, 115 mg sodium, 1.5 g fiber.

Zinc

Your body has about the same amount of zinc as a 4-inch galvanized nail. Getting and maintaining the right amount of zinc is similar to walking a tightrope. It's a fine line between too much and not enough—with hazards for any missteps. Loading up with zinc for more than a week can weaken your immune system, lower your HDL (good) cholesterol and trigger a copper deficiency.

RECOMMENDED INTAKE
RDA (Recommended Dietary Allowance)
Zinc (mg/d)

Life-Stage	Children	Men	Women	Pregnancy	Lactation
1-3 years	3				
4-8 years	5				
9-13 years	8			13	14
14-18 years		11	9	13	14
19-30 years		11	8	11	12
31-50 years		11	8	11	12
51-70 years		11	8		
70+ years		11	8		

Source: The National Academy of Sciences

For optimal health consume 15 to 20 mg per day.

WHAT IS IT?

Unlike other trace minerals, zinc is not stored in the body but acts as a functioning nutrient. Zinc is a party animal—it likes to circulate around and doesn't take time to rest.

Stomach acid is important for the absorption of zinc. Medications or health problems that decrease available stomach acid may limit absorption of zinc. Tumor cells demand zinc for growth and when the supply is plentiful, they thrive. If you have cancer, zinc supplements are usually not recommended. Since zinc is such a circulator, you lose it when your dry skin rubs off or you comb out that "flaky white stuff."

If you substantially increase your calcium intake, you may need more zinc. Vegetarians sometimes have a hard time getting enough zinc because soy foods and whole grains are high in substances that are natural inhibitors of zinc absorption. Zinc found in animal foods, especially red meat, seafood and eggs, is absorbed up to four times more effectively than zinc found in plant foods.

WHY YOU NEED IT

Antioxidant Actions
Teamed up with copper, this mineral helps protect against the damage caused by free radicals.

Hormones
Zinc is needed to make the male hormone testosterone and other essential hormones.

Immune System
Zinc helps put zip in your immune system. Even a mild zinc deficiency can increase your risk of infection.

Metabolism
Zinc plays a role in more than 200 enzymatic reactions in your body. It is critical for the manufacture and stabilization of genetic material. Zinc levels in a pregnant woman are linked to the proper formation of the brain, eyes, heart, bones, lungs, soft palate, lips, kidneys and sex organs of the developing baby.

Skin & Hair
Zinc is needed to help oil glands function. It also helps skin wounds heal by controlling inflammation and speeding regrowth of tissue.

Other Functions
Normal taste and smell senses need plenty of zinc to work properly.

MORE OR LESS?

Increased or decreased nutrient needs should always be discussed with your healthcare professional.

You may need higher than recommended amounts of zinc if you are:
* *Age 70 or older*
* *Alcoholic*
* *Fasting*

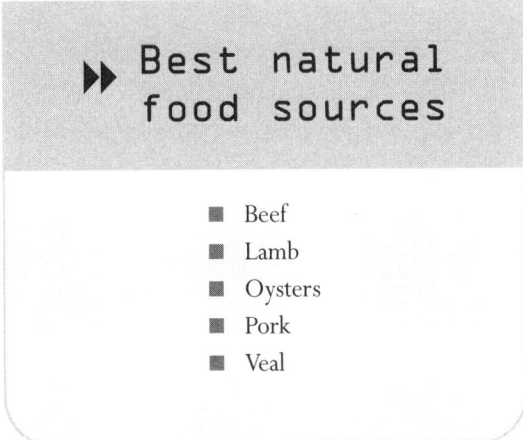

▶▶ Best natural food sources

- Beef
- Lamb
- Oysters
- Pork
- Veal

(Continued...)

- Most fortified ready-to-eat cereals, hot and cold

If You Get Too Little

Lack of zinc may lead to poor night vision, slow wound healing, a decrease in sense of taste and smell, a reduced ability to fight infections and poor development of reproductive organs.

If You Take Too Much

Excess zinc from supplements may cause drowsiness, nausea, vomiting, diarrhea, impaired coordination, restlessness, a weakened immune system, lower HDL (good) cholesterol and decrease copper and iron levels. Minimum toxic dose is 30 mg.

(!) Think twice!

When you are taking zinc supplements, it is especially important that your healthcare professional know if you are also taking copper supplements or tetracycline medication for infections. Wait at least two hours between taking tetracycline and any zinc supplement.

(?) Did you know?

Zinc now added to pennies poses a new risk for stomach ulcers if kids (or anyone) swallow them.

Pesky skin conditions, including dandruff, flaking and psoriasis, speed up zinc losses.

Kitchen Connections

✓ *Enjoy a roast beef sandwich with mustard on rye bread.*
✓ *Add grated gingerroot to pasta dishes and stir-fry.*
✓ *Foods stored in uncoated tin cans may cause less zinc to be available for absorption from food. Buy foods in coated tin cans or choose fresh or frozen forms instead.*

Nutrient Thieves

▶ Milk and eggs reduce zinc absorption. Fiber foods, bran and phytates, found mainly in the outer covering of grains, may also inhibit zinc absorption.

Supplement savvy

Take zinc supplements with food to avoid possible stomach upset. Zinc gluconate and zinc acetate are the most easily absorbed forms of this mineral.

ROAST LEG OF LAMB

Even if you're not aiming for the traces of zinc that lamb offers, this classic method of roasting a leg of lamb will be important to your cooking repertoire.

1 (5- to 6-lb.) leg of lamb, trimmed
4 garlic cloves, halved
3 sprigs fresh rosemary or 1½ teaspoons dried
2 teaspoons lemon-pepper seasoning
½ lemon

❶ Heat oven to 350°F. With sharp-pointed knife, cut 8 slits into lamb surface; insert one piece of garlic into each slit.

❷ Place fatty side up on rack in large roasting pan. Rub with rosemary and lemon-pepper seasoning. Squeeze juice from lemon over meat, rubbing it in. Tuck lemon and rosemary on rack under meat.

❸ Place in oven. Bake 1¼ hours or until internal temperature reaches at least 160°F. Let rest 20 minutes before serving.

8 to 10 servings.
Preparation time: 15 minutes.
Ready to serve: 1 hour, 45 minutes.
Per serving: 285 calories, 12.5 g fat (4.5 g saturated fat), 125 mg cholesterol, 185 mg sodium, 0 g fiber.

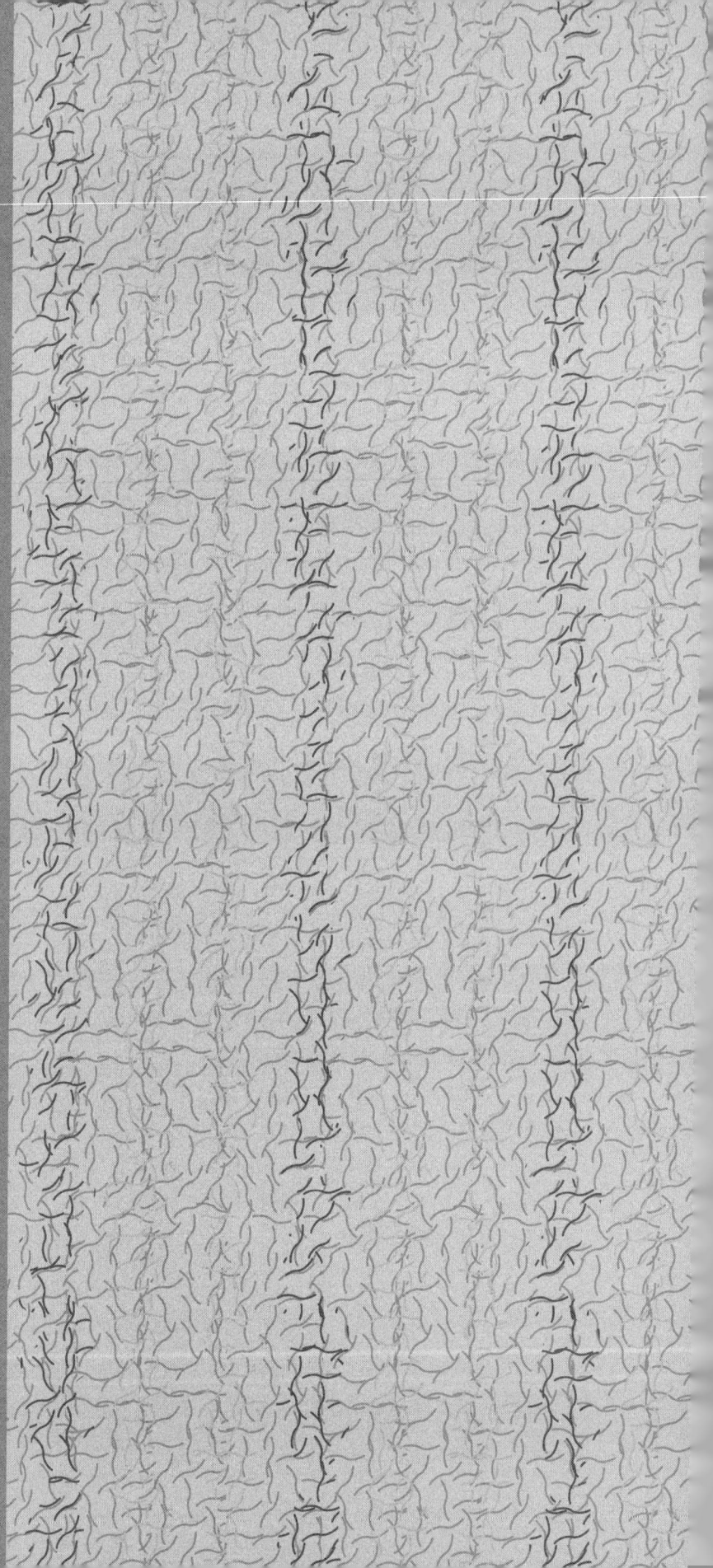

Supplements

N o matter how well you eat, or how well you take care of yourself, sometimes you want to address a specific vitamin or mineral need. That's where supplements enter the nutrition equation. But don't just jump in! You first need to understand the supplement— what it is, the possible benefits, the potential dangers. It's also essential to understand the truth about the claims relating to the supplement. Here are the answers and insights you need.

How to Use This Chapter

*This chapter reviews the wide variety of supplements available
and describes each one in a variety of ways:*

What Is It?
A brief description of each
supplement and its
contents.

Where Is It Found?
When available, food sources
of each supplement are identified, so you won't have to
resort to pills.

Common Doses
Some general guidelines on the
dose you might want to take.

Alpha-Lipoic Acid (ALA)

WHAT IS IT?

Although alpha-lipoic acid (ALA) was thought to be
a vitamin when it was first discovered, subsequent
research determined that it is created in the human
body and thus is not an essential nutrient.

ALA, lipoic acid and thioctic acid are other
names for this vitamin-like antioxidant, sometimes
referred to as the "universal antioxidant" because it
is soluble in both fat and water. ALA is an omega-3
fatty acid. To a limited extent, your body can turn
ALA into eicosapentaenoic acid (EPA)—an omega-3
fatty acid found in fish oil—which, in turn, converts
to 3-series prostaglandins. Prostaglandins are hormone-like substances made in many parts of the
body rather than coming from one organ, as most
hormones do. ALA is capable of regenerating several
other antioxidants back to their active states.

WHERE IS IT FOUND?

Your body makes small amounts of alpha-lipoic acid.
There is limited knowledge about the food sources
of this nutrient; however, foods that contain mitochondria (a specialized component of cells), such as
red meats and yeast, are believed to provide the
most alpha-lipoic acid. Supplements are also
available.

COMMON DOSES

Clinical trials use doses ranging from 150 to 800 mg
per day for up to 2 months. Supplement manufacturers recommend 20 to 50 mg per day on package
labeling.

CLASSIFYING THE CLAIMS

Sound Science	Conflicting Science	Junk Science
Aids diabetics with neuropathy—through injections only, not supplements	Treats glaucoma May slow replication of HIV virus	Enhances athletic performance Slows aging

Think Twice!
Warning notices for potential interactions are noted here.

Did You Know?
With so many myths and miscommunications about the value and use of supplements, it's easy to become confused. Common questions or concerns are addressed here to help you separate fact from fiction.

! Think twice!

Side effects with alpha-lipoic acid are rare but can include skin rash.

Hypoglycemia may develop in diabetics or worsen in those with hypoglycemia.

Individuals who may be deficient in vitamin B1 (such as alcoholics) should take vitamin B1 if they also choose ALA supplements.

? Did you know?

In Germany, alpha-lipoic acid is an approved medical treatment for peripheral neuropathy, a common complication of diabetes. Alpha-lipoic acid speeds the removal of glucose from the bloodstream, by enhancing insulin function and by reducing insulin resistance.

161

Shopping savvy

The only proven benefits of ALA are from intravenous forms and not oral supplements.

Shopping Savvy
Insights and advice on what to look for and how to get the best value when you're shopping for each supplement.

Classifying the Claims
Here, we interpret the benefits of particular supplements. Positive and proven benefits are listed in the **Sound Science** category. When there is no consensus or the research isn't good enough to establish proof positive, those claims will be listed under the **Conflicting Science** heading. The **Junk Science** label means there is no research on benefit claims, or that the research that has been done is of such poor quality that it is inconclusive at best.

5-Hydroxytryptophan (5-HTP)

WHAT IS IT?

A derivative of the amino acid tryptophan, 5-HTP has similar effects and has been shown to improve the quality of sleep by increasing the amount of time spent in deep sleep. The human body uses 5-HTP to make serotonin, an important substance for normal nerve and brain function.

WHERE IS IT FOUND?

Foods do not contain significant amounts of 5-HTP. The human body manufactures 5-HTP from L-tryptophan, a natural amino acid found in many dietary proteins. However, eating food that contains L-tryptophan does not significantly increase 5-HTP levels. Supplemental 5-HTP is naturally derived from the seeds of the *Griffonia simplicifolia*, a West African medicinal plant.

COMMON DOSES

Since there is still concern over potential contamination, 5-HTP is not recommended. (See Did You Know? on page 157.) Common doses range between 50 mg and 900 mg per day.

CLASSIFYING THE CLAIMS

Sound Science	Conflicting Science	Junk Science
Aids insomnia	Treats depression	Aids bipolar (manic-depressive) order
	Treats fibromyalgia	Aids weight loss
	Treats insomnia	Aids Parkinson's disease
	Treats migraines	

! Think twice!

Do not take 5-HTP with antidepressants, weight-control drugs or other serotonin-modifying medications. The combination of drugs increases the rate of side effects.

Individuals with liver disease might not be able to regulate 5-HTP adequately, and those suffering from autoimmune diseases may be more sensitive to 5-HTP.

Side effects many include gastrointestinal upset, headache, sleepiness, muscle pain and anxiety.

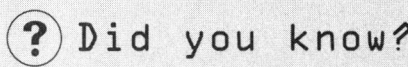

? Did you know?

A substance known as "Peak X" has been found in low concentrations in several over-the-counter 5-HTP preparations that some researchers think may be linked to toxicity. FDA scientists have confirmed the presence of impurities in some 5-HTP products.

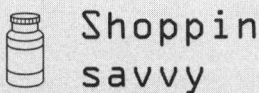

Shopping savvy

Sometimes 5-HTP is combined with herbs or other ingredients that may not be safe or necessary. Check the label to be sure you know what you are buying.

Do not take supplements of 5-HTP for more than 8 to 12 weeks without being monitored by a healthcare professional.

Acidophilus

WHAT IS IT?

Acidophilus is one of many strains of the lactic acid bacteria found normally in the human intestinal tract, mouth and vagina. Though it has been thought of for hundreds of years as a health food, scientific research first began in the 1900s. Acidophilus is now recognized as one of the most beneficial of all intestinal bacteria.

WHERE IS IT FOUND?

Acidophilus is found in some yogurt, kefir and other dairy foods. It's also added as a supplement to some beverages. You can purchase acidophilus in tablet or powder form.

COMMON DOSES

Some experts recommend 1 billion to 10 billion cells per day. Acidophilus has been on the market for many decades in yogurt and other dairy products, with no reported side effects.

CLASSIFYING THE CLAIMS

Sound Science	Conflicting Science	Junk Science
Treats antibiotic-associated diarrhea	Prevents vaginal yeast infections Improves digestibility of dairy products Lowers cholesterol	Treats vaginal yeast infections with direct application of yogurt products

(!) Think twice!

Don't self-treat your first vaginal yeast infection with acidophilus. Seek the advice of a healthcare professional.

Though acidophilus is safe for children with diarrhea, be sure to seek advice from a healthcare professional if severe diarrhea lasts longer than 24 hours.

(?) Did you know?

Research shows that it is best to buy products that have a single strain of acidophilus and not the mixed variety. Single strains tend to be more effective.

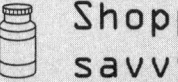 Shopping savvy

Acidophilus comes in powders, tablets, capsules or added to foods. Improper handling and storage of acidophilus supplements can kill or reduce the number of live bacteria. Keep acidophilus foods in the refrigerator; do not freeze. Store powder or tablet supplements in a cool, dry place.

Alpha-Lipoic Acid (ALA)

WHAT IS IT?

Although alpha-lipoic acid (ALA) was thought to be a vitamin when it was first discovered, subsequent research determined that it is created in the human body and thus is not an essential nutrient.

ALA, lipoic acid and thioctic acid are other names for this vitamin-like antioxidant, sometimes referred to as the "universal antioxidant" because it is soluble in both fat and water. ALA is an omega-3 fatty acid. To a limited extent, your body can turn ALA into eicosapentaenoic acid (EPA)—an omega-3 fatty acid found in fish oil—which, in turn, converts to 3-series prostaglandins. Prostaglandins are hormone-like substances made in many parts of the body rather than coming from one organ, as most hormones do. ALA is capable of regenerating several other antioxidants back to their active states.

WHERE IS IT FOUND?

Your body makes small amounts of alpha-lipoic acid. There is limited knowledge about the food sources of this nutrient; however, foods that contain mitochondria (a specialized component of cells), such as red meats and yeast, are believed to provide the most alpha-lipoic acid. Supplements are also available.

COMMON DOSES

Clinical trials use doses ranging from 150 to 800 mg per day for up to 2 months. Supplement manufacturers recommend 20 to 50 mg per day on package labeling.

CLASSIFYING THE CLAIMS

Sound Science	Conflicting Science	Junk Science
Aids diabetics with neuropathy—through injections only, not supplements	Treats glaucoma May slow replication of HIV virus	Enhances athletic performance Slows aging

! Think twice!

Side effects with alpha-lipoic acid are rare but can include skin rash.

Hypoglycemia may develop in diabetics or worsen in those with hypoglycemia.

Individuals who may be deficient in vitamin B1 (such as alcoholics) should take vitamin B1 if they also choose ALA supplements.

? Did you know?

In Germany, alpha-lipoic acid is an approved medical treatment for peripheral neuropathy, a common complication of diabetes. Alpha-lipoic acid speeds the removal of glucose from the bloodstream, by enhancing insulin function and by reducing insulin resistance.

 ## Shopping savvy

The only proven benefits of ALA are from intravenous forms and not oral supplements.

Arginine

WHAT IS IT?

Arginine is a nonessential amino acid that helps stimulate growth hormones and your immune system. While it's true that arginine can stimulate the secretion of growth hormones, it must be taken in massive amounts—more than can be found in supplements—to do so.

WHERE IS IT FOUND?

Most foods that contain protein also contain arginine, including meat, fish, nuts, whole grains and chocolate.

COMMON DOSES

No safe dosage has been established. Typical products provide 500 mg to 25 g in tablet, capsule or powder form.

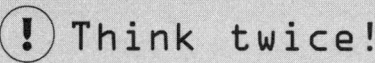

⚠ Think twice!

High intakes of arginine may interfere with metabolism of other amino acids.

People with herpes simplex virus should not take supplemental arginine; because arginine is required for the virus to replicate, excess levels may make outbreaks worse.

CLASSIFYING THE CLAIMS

Sound Science	Conflicting Science	Junk Science
None	Heals wounds and burns	Builds muscle
	Enhances immune function	Increases growth hormone
		Aids weight loss

Shopping savvy

Single amino acid supplements are not recommended.

? Did you know?

As far back as 1978, arginine (along with the amino acids cystine, treonine, tyrosine, leucine, methioine, phenylalanine and valine) was investigated by a scientific panel and was found to be worthless as a weight-loss aid.

Bee Pollen

WHAT IS IT?

Bees keep busy bringing nectar and pollen to the hive—it's their full-time, lifelong job. They collect the pollen on their body hairs, place it in "pollen baskets" on their legs, then carry it back to the hive to be deposited in the honey cells.

WHERE IS IT FOUND?

Bee pollen is sold in tablet and capsule form.

COMMON DOSES

No safe dose has been established. Manufacturers commonly recommend ½ to 1 teaspoon of bee pollen per day.

⚠ Think twice!

Eating "nature's most perfect food" can make you sick. Bee pollen can cause life-threatening allergic reactions in some people, even though it's often promoted as an allergy cure. Some early warning signs include numbness or tingling on your lips or in your mouth. If you have any reactions to eating bee pollen, go directly to the closest emergency room.

CLASSIFYING THE CLAIMS

Sound Science	Conflicting Science	Junk Science
		Nature's perfect food
		Treats infection
		Treats allergies

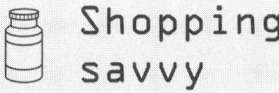 Shopping savvy

Bee pollen is sold in capsules and is often added as a supplement to smoothies.

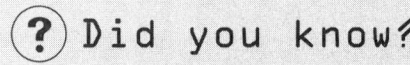 Did you know?

Bee pollen has only trace amounts of the vitamins and minerals it boasts, and many of these nutrients are in a form that is unavailable to the human digestive system.

Carnitine

WHAT IS IT?

Carnitine is a nonessential amino acid that plays a key role in fatty acid metabolism. It's considered nonessential because your body can make its own when you don't get enough from foods you eat.

WHERE IS IT FOUND?

Food sources of carnitine include red meats and dairy products. Fruits, vegetables, grains and eggs also contain tiny amounts of carnitine. Almost all carnitine in the body is found in bones and the heart muscle.

COMMON DOSES

No safe dosage has been established. Manufacturers recommend 2 to 4 g of carnitine, divided into 2 or 3 doses.

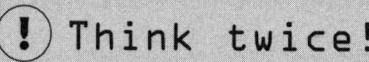 ! Think twice!

High intakes may interfere with metabolism of other amino acids.

More than 6 g per day may cause nausea and diarrhea.

CLASSIFYING THE CLAIMS

Sound Science	Conflicting Science	Junk Science
Treats antibiotic-associated diarrhea	Slows onset of Alzheimer's Enhances immune function Improves heart functioning	Enhances athletic performance Aids weight loss

Shopping savvy

Single amino acid supplements are not recommended.

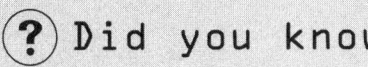 ## Did you know?

Individuals with certain kidney or liver disorders may have a special need for carnitine and, therefore, it becomes an essential amino acid for these groups.

Carotenoids

WHAT ARE THEY?

Carotenoids are a group of about 600 nutrients; they are neither vitamins nor phytochemicals. Carotenes are converted in the body to vitamin A. The most widely studied carotenoid is beta-carotene. Other key carotenes include lycopene, lutein and zeaxanthin.

The exact way that carotenoids work to promote health is not known, but it's thought they protect cells from oxidative damage. Experts believe that carotenoids work best as a team along with phyto-chemicals and vitamins.

WHERE ARE THEY FOUND?

Beta-carotene
* Carrots
* Pumpkin
* Squash
* Sweet potatoes
* Leafy greens

Lutein and Zeaxanthin
* Leafy greens
* Broccoli
* Zucchini
* Corn

Lycopene
* Tomatoes
* Tomato products (ketchup and sauces)
* Watermelon
* Pink grapefruit

CLASSIFYING THE CLAIMS

Sound Science	Conflicting Science	Junk Science
Reduces risk of cataracts (lutein and zeaxanthin)	Reduces the risk of cancer (lycopene)	
Reduces risk of macular degeneration (lutein and zeaxanthin)	Reduces risk of heart disease (lycopene)	
	Treats cystic fibrosis (Beta-carotene)	

Common Doses

The amount commonly found in supplements is 10 to 15 mg per day. It's so much more enjoyable to get carotenoids from foods.

Chitosan

WHAT IS IT?

Chitosan is derived from chitin, a polysaccharide found in the exoskeleton of shellfish such as shrimp, lobster and crabs. It's made of the indigestible fiber from the shells. When chemically treated, chitin becomes chitosan, which has some ability to bind fat and limit fat absorption.

WHERE IS IT FOUND?

Chitosan is made from crushed shrimp, crab and/or lobster shells.

COMMON DOSES

There is no safe dose established for chitosan. Manufacturers recommend 400 mg with each meal.

CLASSIFYING THE CLAIMS		
Sound Science	**Conflicting Science**	**Junk Science**
		Fat magnet/burns fat
		Lowers cholesterol
		Lowers high blood pressure
		Reduces risk of heart attack
		Reduces risk of cancer

! Think twice!

If you are allergic to shellfish, you should avoid chitosan supplements.

 ## Shopping savvy

Taking the manufacturers' recommended dose of 400 mg per meal would block absorption of less than 5 grams of fat over the course of a day. That would save you just 45 calories. At this rate, it would take you 77 days to lose one pound if you didn't make any other changes—not great results.

? Did you know?

Because crab and lobster shells are a natural substance that can't be patented, there is little financial incentive to conduct extensive studies. As with other products, manufacturers can label it a dietary supplement and go to market without FDA approval or review.

Chlorophyll

WHAT IS IT?

Chlorophyll is the substance responsible for the green color in plants. It has been used historically to control bad breath and treat infected wounds.

WHERE IS IT FOUND?

Food sources of chlorophyll include dark green leafy vegetables, algae, spirulina, chlorella, wheat grass and barley grass.

COMMON DOSES

Package recommendations suggest 100 mg, 1 to 3 times a day. For bad breath, label directions say to mix 1 teaspoon powder with 4 ounces water, then swish and swallow or spit out.

(!) Think twice!

Chlorophyll supplements may cause some people to experience nausea or diarrhea. You can minimize this effect by taking supplements with food.

CLASSIFYING THE CLAIMS

Sound Science	Conflicting Science	Junk Science
Controls bad breath	Anti-inflammatory agent	Detoxifies cancer-causing substances

Shopping savvy

Supplements of chlorophyll are available as powders, capsules, tablets and beverages.

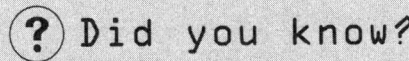 ## Did you know?

Chlorophyll has no nutritional benefits beyond what is traditionally available in vegetable foods. Unless you want an expensive, natural breath freshener, spend your money on produce and brush your teeth more often.

173

Cholestin

What Is It?

Cholestin comes from Monascus, a strain of red yeast that is sometimes used in Chinese cooking. For centuries, it has been used in traditional Chinese medicine to help maintain a healthy heart and circulatory system. Cholestin contains the natural ingredient mevinolin. This substance is similar to the statin drugs—such as Zocor, Pravachol and Lipitor—that doctors prescribe for high cholesterol. Cholestin blocks the action of an enzyme in the liver that triggers cholesterol production. It can be purchased without a prescription as an over-the-counter dietary supplement at one-fifth the cost.

Where Is It Found?

Red yeast rice is commonly consumed in Asian countries as part of the traditional cuisine. It's used as a spice or seasoning for foods such as Peking duck.

Common Doses

Red yeast rice is supplied in capsules of varying size. The typical dosage recommendation is 1,200 mg daily, divided into two doses. Do not exceed 2,400 mg daily.

CLASSIFYING THE CLAIMS		
Sound Science	**Conflicting Science**	**Junk Science**
Lowers high cholesterol		

! Think twice!

In very high doses, the mevinolin in red yeast rice has been known to damage the liver. Do not take it if you have liver disease, are in danger of developing it, or consume more than two alcoholic beverages a day.

It's best to stop using red yeast rice during any serious infection.

If you develop any muscle pain or tenderness, discontinue the product immediately and check with your healthcare provider.

Do not combine cholestin with prescription cholesterol-lowering drugs.

? Did you know?

The FDA has ruled in favor of drug companies who wanted to ban over-the-counter sales of cholestin because the statin drugs require a prescription and cholestin has many of the same side effects as the statin drugs.

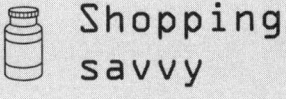 Shopping savvy

Take with food to reduce the risk of digestive disturbance.

CoQ-10

WHAT IS IT?

Each of your cells contains a miniature power factory called the mitochondrion. This is where the energy your body needs is made. CoQ-10 helps regulate the electrical currents that fuel this factory. Imagine a string of holiday lights: If one of the bulbs doesn't work, the others go out too. It's CoQ-10's job to get in there and replace any defective or empty sockets so the system keeps functioning. Coenzyme Q10 (CoQ-10) is an essential component of the energy-producing parts of your body's cells.

WHERE IS IT FOUND?

Ubiquinone, or CoQ-10, is found in every cell of every plant and animal on earth. Meat, poultry, fish and dairy foods are the main sources in most diets.

COMMON DOSES

It takes a minimum of eight weeks to produce any noticeable results. Most people take about 150 to 300 mg per day.

(!) Think twice!

You may experience some mild gastrointestinal upset.

If you take more than 600 mg per day, you should have routine checks to monitor renal function.

CLASSIFYING THE CLAIMS

Sound Science	Conflicting Science	Junk Science
Antioxidant actions	Enhances heart function	Improves athletic performance
	Enhances immune system	Slows aging
	Aids congestive heart failure	Aids weight loss
		Treats or prevents cancer

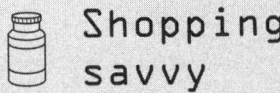 Shopping savvy

Look for the newer soluble form of CoQ-10. There is limited evidence that it is absorbed more efficiently than other forms and, therefore, lower doses would be needed.

(?) Did you know?

The Japanese were the first to take CoQ-10 supplements. There is lots of exciting evidence that this supplement may play a significant role in helping those with heart disease. Currently, research trials have only supplemented people with CoQ-10 for one year. There are no long-term studies that guarantee the safety and benefits of CoQ-10 over the long run.

Creatine

WHAT IS IT?

Creatine is found naturally in animal muscle tissue. Its name come from the Greek word for flesh. Creatine monohydrate is converted to creatine phosphate and stored in the muscle cells until it's needed to make chemical energy.

WHERE IS IT FOUND?

Food sources of creatine include meat, poultry and fish. If plenty of creatine isn't available from the foods you eat, the liver and kidneys easily make it from a few amino acids (arginine, glycine and methioine).

COMMON DOSES

Manufacturers recommend 20 to 25 grams per day during a weeklong "loading phase," in divided doses of 5 grams taken 4 or 5 times a day. This dose is tapered to 2 to 10 grams daily during the "maintenance phase." Extra water when supplementing with creatine is essential to prevent dehydration.

CLASSIFYING THE CLAIMS

Sound Science	Conflicting Science	Junk Science
Promotes weight gain Benefits athletes only during high intensity, intermittent exercise	Enhances heart function Allows athletes to train at higher intensity Combats muscle loss associated with muscular dystrophy and ALS	Improves athletic performance Slows aging Delays exercise fatigue

! Think twice!

Creatine is definitely not recommended for young athletes.

Some creatine users report increased muscle cramping (especially during exercise in high heat), nausea and other gastrointestinal disturbances.

Creatine supplementation, in the doses commonly used, results in urine concentrations that are 90 times greater than normal. Since the kidneys filter creatine there is the potential for significant kidney damage or disease with long-term use.

No long-term safety studies have been done and most research is limited to just a few weeks of observation of creatine's effects on the body.

Caffeine may interfere with any potential ergogenic (athletic performance enhancement) effects provided by creatine.

? Did you know?

When certain athletes supplement with extra amounts of creatine, their muscles can produce more quick energy, but only in highly explosive activities or those with quick repetitive movements. If you need to bat a ball, thrust heavy weights or tackle your opponent to the ground, you might gain a competitive edge with creatine. If you're an endurance athlete, such as a distance runner, swimmer or triathlete, creatine won't help. Use of creatine by nonathletes is senseless.

Shopping savvy

Before you take creatine supplements—and they are not recommended—have baseline kidney and liver function tests performed by your healthcare provider.

Avoid creatine supplements that also contain caffeine.

Dehydroepiandrosterone (DHEA)

WHAT IS IT?

DHEA is a hormone that helps regulate sexual maturation. When you wake each morning, the adrenal glands nestled on top of your kidneys release a form of DHEA into your bloodstream. As it merges into body tissues, DHEA is converted into tiny amounts of the sex hormones testosterone and estrogen. Normal DHEA levels increase sharply at puberty, peak during early adulthood and then gradually diminish until there's practically none left.

WHERE IS IT FOUND?

DHEA is a hormone and is not a part of food.

COMMON DOSAGE

DHEA is not recommended at any dose.

CLASSIFYING THE CLAIMS		
Sound Science	Conflicting Science	Junk Science
Speeds spread of prostate, breast and endometrial cancers		Slows aging Enhances immune system Aids weight loss

! Think twice!

DHEA supplementation alters levels of other hormones and the effects of this action are not fully documented.

DHEA may increase levels of testosterone in males and increase risk of prostate cancer.

In women, excess DHEA may increase growth of facial hair, increase acne, deepen the voice and cause menstrual irregularities.

DHEA also has some estrogenic activity that may increase the risk of hormone-stimulated cancers.

? Did you know?

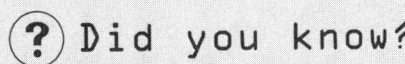

The FDA banned over-the-counter sales of DHEA in 1985 because of its potentially harmful side effects. Since then, it's reappeared in exactly the same form as a "dietary supplement," which, of course, doesn't require FDA approval.

Shopping savvy

Human hormones are powerful chemicals. Do-it-yourself DHEA hormone therapy is just plain D-U-M-B.

Fish Oils—EPA and DHA

WHAT ARE THEY?

Fish oil contains EPA (eicosapentanoic acid) and DHA (docosahexanoic acid); both are omega-3 fatty acids. These long-chained fatty acids have been shown to have many positive effects. As a part of the cell membranes, fatty acids help form a physical barrier to keep out viruses, bacteria and other foreign molecules. They also regulate the traffic of substances in and out of the cells. Because we tend to eat lots of processed foods that are higher in omega-6 fatty acids, nature's balance is upset. The typical American diet provides low amounts of omega-3 fatty acids and this has been linked to the increase in many of today's common chronic diseases.

CLASSIFYING THE CLAIMS

Sound Science	Conflicting Science	Junk Science
Anti-inflammatory	Decreases atherosclerosis	Treats asthma
Enhances immune function	Treats depression	Treats diabetes
Treats Crohn's disease	Lowers risk of cancer	Treats migraines
Lowers high triglycerides	Treats schizophrenia	Treats osteoporosis
Helps premature infants with catch-up growth	Treats attention deficit hyperactive disorder	
	Lowers high blood pressure	
	Treats kidney disease	

WHERE ARE THEY FOUND?

EPA and DHA are found in mackerel, salmon, herring, sardines, sable fish (black cod), anchovies, albacore tuna and wild game. Two to three fish servings per week are suggested. Cod liver oil contains large amounts of EPA and DHA. To a very limited extent, omega-3 fatty acids from vegetable sources, such as flaxseed oil, can convert to EPA. There are also EPA- and DHA-fortified foods such as eggs, margarine, milk, yogurt and bread—check the label.

COMMON DOSES

Although there is no set limit for omega-3 fatty acids, the FDA suggests that up to 3 grams are safe. Most of the research with fish oil has given people with a variety of health conditions at least 3 grams of EPA plus DHA—an amount that may require 10 grams of fish oil, because most fish oil contains only 18 percent EPA and 12 percent DHA.

(!) Think twice!

Check with your healthcare provider before taking more than 3 or 4 grams of fish oil daily. Elevations in blood sugar and cholesterol levels may occur in some individuals who take these supplements.

Fish oils act as blood thinners, so you should not take them with any anticoagulant medications or if you have blood-clotting problems. Some people taking supplements are prone to nosebleeds.

Because of its very high levels of vitamin A and vitamin D, pregnant women should not take cod liver oil.

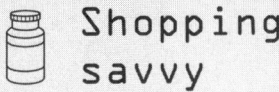

Shopping savvy

Fish oil is easily damaged by oxygen, so a few milligrams or IUs of vitamin E should be included in all fish oil supplements. In addition, people who supplement with fish oil should take additional vitamin E supplements (50 to 100 IUs daily) to protect EPA and DHA within the body from oxidative damage.

Buy capsules labeled "distilled" or "molecularly distilled," which ensures that they are virtually free of PCBs, mercury and lead, which tend to accumulate in some fish. A cholesterol-free designation usually indicates distillation too.

Store fish oil capsules and supplements in the refrigerator.

Some people who supplement several grams of fish oil will experience gastrointestinal upset and burp a "fishy" smell.

The enteric-coated free fatty acid form has been reported not to cause the gastrointestinal symptoms that often result from taking regular fish oil supplements.

The health benefits for individuals with Crohn's disease have been reported with a special enteric-coated, free fatty acid form of EPA/DHA from fish oil.

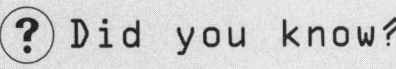

(?) Did you know?

If you choose fish oil capsules, remember you are also swallowing fat grams and calories.

Flaxseed

WHAT IS IT?

Flaxseed comes from plants that have been cultivated in Central Asia for more than 5,000 years. Flaxseed is about 35 percent fat and is a rich source of omega-3 fatty acids and lignins (a type of fiber). Flaxseed oil contains 100 to 800 times more plant lignins than other common seed oils. Lignins have special properties that work as antioxidants, help slow tumor growth and have anti-inflammatory properties. Like most vegetable oils, flaxseed also contains linoleic acid, an essential fatty acid.

WHERE IS IT FOUND?

Flaxseed and flaxseed oil are found in most supermarkets. Some margarine is made with flaxseed oil.

Some breads and cereals may contain added flaxseed.

COMMON DOSES

A common recommendation is 1 tablespoon per day. You can add flaxseed oil as a dressing on salads or drizzled over vegetables. Remember that flaxseed, like all oils, is high in fat and calorie content. Flaxseed oil provides 140 calories and 14 grams of fat per tablespoon.

CLASSIFYING THE CLAIMS

Sound Science	Conflicting Science	Junk Science
Treats constipation	Lowers high cholesterol	Aids ulcerative colitis
Antioxidant actions	May increase or decrease risk for some cancers	
Anti-inflammatory		

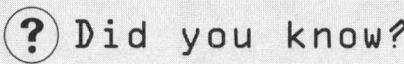

! Think twice!

Taking more than 4 tablespoons of flaxseed oil per day may have a laxative effect.

Flaxseed supplements may increase bleeding time and are not recommended if you are undergoing surgery or have a disorder of blood clotting.

? Did you know?

Don't use flaxseed oil for high temperature cooking such as popping corn or stir-frying. The beneficial ingredients break down at high temperatures. Store your flax oil refrigerated in an airtight, opaque container.

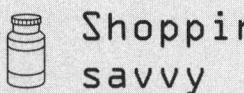

Shopping savvy

Flaxseeds must be ground before adding to breads, muffins or salads. Whole flaxseed can't be digested by the human gastrointestinal tract unless ground or chopped first.

Fructo-Oligosaccharides (FOS)

WHAT ARE THEY?

Fructo-oligosaccharides (FOS) are naturally occurring carbohydrates that cannot be digested or absorbed by humans but support the growth of bifidobacteria, one of the beneficial bacterial strains. As a result, some doctors recommend FOS to all patients who are supplementing bifidobacteria. (For further information about bifidobacteria and probiotics, see pages 206–207.)

WHERE ARE THEY FOUND?

The most common food sources of FOS are wheat, barley, rye, onions, bananas, tomatoes, garlic, leeks, chicory root and Jerusalem artichokes. The amount of FOS in any of these foods is still low. It would take 16 tomatoes or 13 bananas to get just one gram of FOS. Supplementation is a practical way to attain the 1 to 4 grams of FOS recommended daily.

COMMON DOSAGE

Several trials have used 8 grams per day. However, a review of the research has suggested that 4 grams per day appears to be enough to significantly increase the amount of bifidobacteria in the stomach.

CLASSIFYING THE CLAIMS

Sound Science	Conflicting Science	Junk Science
Reduces some types of diarrhea	Prevents constipation Increases calcium absorption	Lowers cholesterol Treats IBD

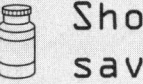 ## Shopping savvy

A common daily recommendation is 1 to 4 grams of FOS, usually from fortified food supplements. When you first start taking FOS, gas, cramps and bloating may occur as the bad bacteria dies off and the good bacteria flourishes in your digestive system. Starting with a lower, divided dose can help alleviate these side effects.

(?) Did you know?

Some proponents of probiotics claim that it's better to increase your own strain of bacteria than to introduce new colonies of bacteria.

Gamma Butyrolactone (GBL)

What Is It?

When taken orally, GBL is converted in the body to gamma hydroxybutyrate or GHB. A very potent unapproved drug, GHB is currently being investigated under the supervision of doctors for the treatment of narcolepsy. Because of its serious side effects, GHB should not be taken unless in the context of these FDA approved investigations. GBL is also known by the chemical names 2(3H)-furanone dihydro; butyrolactone; gamma-butyrolactone; 4-butyrolactone; dihydro-2(3H)-furanone; 4-butanolide; 2(3H)-furanone, dihydro; tetrahydro-2-furanone; and butyrolactone gamma.

Where Is It Found?

GBL is an ingredient in a variety of liquid and powder supplements. Some popular supplements that include GBL are Blue Nitro, Revivarant, Gamma G and Remforce.

Common Doses

GBL is not recommended in any dose.

CLASSIFYING THE CLAIMS

Sound Science	Conflicting Science	Junk Science
		Builds muscle
		Enhances sex drive
		Treats insomnia

! Think twice!

Many people have gotten sick from GBL supplements and it's been blamed for at least one death. Symptoms include seizures, slowed breathing and a slowed heart rate. About one-third of those who reported problems became unconscious or comatose.

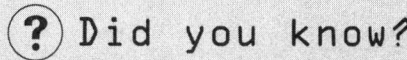

? Did you know?

In January 1999, the FDA asked all companies distributing or producing products with GBL to recall them.

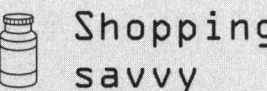

Shopping savvy

No one should take GBL. The FDA and the Justice Department have ongoing criminal enforcement actions against those who market GBL products. The FDA advises anyone in possession of these products to dispose of them immediately.

Glucosamine

WHAT IS IT?

Glucosamine is an amino-sugar that gives cartilage strength and rigidity. Cartilage is the smooth, rubbery stuff that acts like a shock absorber at the ends of your bones. You've probably seen it at the top of a chicken or turkey drumstick. This cartilage protects your bones from rubbing together and wearing away. Overactive enzymes that break down the tissue cause wear and tear on the cartilage. Recent research shows that glucosamine may stimulate the growth of new cartilage and help fend off the effects of harmful enzymes.

WHERE IS IT FOUND?

There are no food sources of glucosamine. Glucosamine sulfate supplements come primarily from crab, lobster or shrimp shells. Another less helpful version, glucosamine chondroitin, is extracted primarily from cow trachea cartilage.

COMMON DOSES

There is no established safe dosage for glucosamine. Manufacturers and clinical trials studying glucosamine usually provide a total of 1500 mg per day, divided into three doses of 500 mg each.

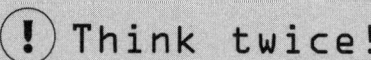

(!) Think twice!

Because of its animal source, vegetarians may not want to use glucosamine.

There is the possibility that individuals allergic to shellfish may have a reaction to glucosamine.

CLASSIFYING THE CLAIMS

Sound Science	Conflicting Science	Junk Science
Treats osteoarthritis		Treats rheumatoid arthritis

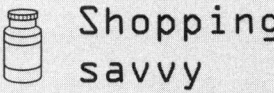 ## Shopping savvy

Glucosamine hydrochloride or glucosamine sulfate are the forms used in most research—look for either of these on the ingredient label.

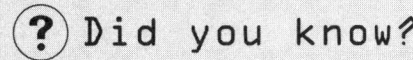 ## Did you know?

Veterinarians have been using glucosamine since 1992 to successfully treat osteoarthritis in racehorses, farm animals and pets.

Glycerol

WHAT IS IT?

Glycerol is a core part of triglycerides (fats) and phospholipids found in your body. It is made by your body and stored in fatty tissue and found in your bloodstream. In the liver, glycerol can be converted into glucose.

WHERE IS IT FOUND?

Glycerol is not a normal part of foods. It is used as an additive in many processed foods, medications and skin products.

COMMON DOSES

Athletes commonly use 1 gram of glycerol in the form of glycerate per kilogram (2.2 pounds) of body weight mixed with a large volume of water. This mixture is then consumed 1 to 1½ hours before strenuous exercise. No safe or recommended dose is known.

(!) Think twice!

Because glycerol can cause fluid retention, it should be avoided by anyone with edema, congestive heart failure, kidney disease or high blood pressure.

Side effects may include headache and blurred vision.

CLASSIFYING THE CLAIMS

Sound Science	Conflicting Science	Junk Science
		Superhydrator
		Increases ability to exercise in hot, humid weather

Shopping savvy

Glycerol is available in drugstores as glycerin or glycerine in oral and topical varieties. It is also sold as glycerate in powdered form or can be added to sports beverages.

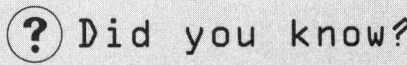 ## (?) Did you know?

Glycerol is sometimes used to help lower pressure in the head of individuals suffering stroke, meningitis and encephalitis during hospitalization. Sometimes glycerol is used as a medication to help reduce pressure in the eyes in glaucoma. Glycerol tends to cause fluid retention everywhere in the body except in the head and eyes.

Kelp

WHAT IS IT?

Kelp is one of several brown-colored seaweed species called Laminaria. This sea vegetable is a concentrated source of minerals including iodine, potassium, magnesium, calcium and iron. Dried kelp is a source of iodine, and has been used medicinally since the beginning of the 19th century.

WHERE IS IT FOUND?

This long-stemmed seaweed is found on the North Atlantic coast. It's most commonly sold in health food stores.

COMMON DOSES

No safe dosage has been established. Since the introduction of iodized salt, additional sources of iodine, such as kelp, are unnecessary.

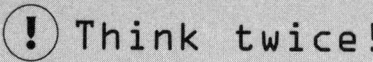

! Think twice!

Be careful about the amount you take. Doses of iodine in excess of 150 micrograms a day can induce or worsen an overactive thyroid gland.

Warning signs of excessive thyroid stimulation include thyroid enlargement, rapid heartbeat, palpitations, nervousness, agitation, increased sweating, fatigue, weakness, insomnia, increased appetite and weight loss.

Severe allergic reactions, although rare, are also a possible risk.

CLASSIFYING THE CLAIMS		
Sound Science	**Conflicting Science**	**Junk Science**
	Prevents iodine deficiency	Treats thyroid disease

Shopping savvy

Iodine supplements are available in tablet, capsule and liquid forms. It is often combined with potassium.

(?) Did you know?

It's not safe to harvest your own kelp from the wild. It may be contaminated with heavy metals or toxins from industrial waste or farm and garden runoff.

L-Tryptophan

What Is It?

L-tryptophan is an essential amino acid and is not normally found in the human diet by itself. It functions as a metabolic precursor to serotonin—a chemical messenger in your brain and central nervous system.

L-tryptophan is perhaps the most infamous of all supplements. Pills containing this amino acid were marketed as a solution for people with insomnia in the 1970s. More than 1,200 individuals who took tryptophan developed a painful connective tissue and blood disease called eosinophilia-myalgia syndrome. At least 38 people died from exposure to a contaminant in the supplement. In 1990, the FDA pulled L-tryptophan off store shelves.

Where Is It Found?

L-tryptophan is found in high protein foods like meats, fish, poultry, eggs, dairy products and nuts.

Common Doses

This supplement is not safe at any dose.

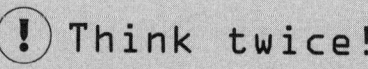

(!) Think twice!

Eosinophilia-myalgia syndrome is a rare and sometimes fatal disorder linked with tryptophan supplements.

Other possible side effects include nausea, constipation, gas and reduced sex drive.

Classifying the Claims

Sound Science	Conflicting Science	Junk Science
Treats insomnia	Mood enhancer	

Shopping savvy

You can no longer purchase tryptophan in the United States, but 5-HTP—a supplement that contains a form of tryptophan—is available though still not recommended.

(?) Did you know?

Dietary tryptophan has to compete with other amino acids for entry into the brain after you eat a high-protein meal. After a high-carbohydrate meal, insulin causes the competing amino acids to enter the muscles. This is why meals with lots of carbohydrates (and tryptophan) cause you to feel drowsy while high-protein meals don't.

Lecithin

WHAT IS IT?

Lecithin is a natural compound that includes choline, inositol, phosphorus and various fatty acids. It is found throughout the body, and is available in a variety of foods as well as in natural and synthetic supplements. Lecithin is about 13 percent choline by weight. Your body makes all the lecithin you need. However, some groups are at risk for deficiency, including infants, pregnant women, those with cirrhosis of the liver and people on tube or IV feedings. By promoting the normal processing of fat and cholesterol, lecithin may protect against hardening of the arteries and heart disease.

WHERE IS IT FOUND?

Eggs, red meat, peanut butter, cabbage, cauliflower, lentils, green beans, soybeans and oranges are all good food sources of lecithin.

COMMON DOSES

There is no RDA for lecithin. Two tablespoons daily is the usual dosage.

CLASSIFYING THE CLAIMS		
Sound Science	**Conflicting Science**	**Junk Science**
	Removes/reduces fat buildup in arteries	Enhances athletic performance Slows onset of Alzheimer's disease Improves memory and concentration

! Think twice!

Excessive doses can cause dizziness, nausea and vomiting.

Amounts over 700 grams per day may lead to urinary incontinence, diarrhea and fishy body odor.

If you are taking nicotinic acid (a form of niacin) to lower your cholesterol, you may be advised to take lecithin as a way of boosting your choline intake. High levels of niacin tend to deplete the choline in your system.

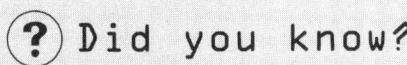

? Did you know?

Lecithin is used as an emulsifier in many processed foods such as mayonnaise, ice cream and salad dressing.

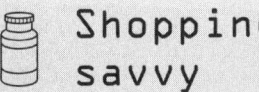

Shopping savvy

Most lecithin supplements are made from either eggs or soy products. You don't really need extra. If you think you do, just eat the real thing.

Melatonin

What Is It?

Melatonin is a naturally occurring hormone that helps regulate sleep. Cued by nightfall, melatonin production begins at dusk and halts each morning as the sun rises. Your pineal gland (found in the brain) is the master controller of this rhythmic hormone that sets your sleeping and waking schedule. If you happen to live in a northern latitude where winter darkness extends beyond your normal wake-up time, you know melatonin's strong grip. Your body correctly senses it's still nighttime when it's dark outside, and convinces you to stay in bed.

Where Is It Found?

Only tiny amounts of melatonin are found in plant foods. No one food contains much, but rice, barley, sweet corn and oats have the highest concentration.

Common Doses

Most manufacturers recommend taking from 1 to 3 mg of melatonin approximately 20 minutes before bedtime. Controlled release formulations should be taken 2 hours before going to bed.

CLASSIFYING THE CLAIMS

Sound Science	Conflicting Science	Junk Science
	Treats insomnia	Reduces risk of cancer
	Reduces jet lag	Slows aging
		Lowers high cholesterol
		Lowers high blood pressure

Think twice!

Do not take melatonin if you have an autoimmune disease such as rheumatoid arthritis, any condition that affects your lymphatic system, AIDS, osteoarthritis, depression or any other emotional disorder, diabetes, epilepsy, heart disease, leukemia, multiple sclerosis or serious allergies.

Couples who are trying to conceive a baby should avoid this hormone.

Melatonin is not recommended for use in children or teenagers.

Take melatonin only at bedtime. Do not drive or operate machinery after taking a dose.

If you develop a headache, rash or upset stomach, or find that your normal sleeping patterns are disrupted, stop taking melatonin and check with your doctor.

Check with your healthcare provider before combining melatonin with beta-blockers, ibuprofen or steroids.

Do not take melatonin supplements during pregnancy or while breastfeeding.

Shopping savvy

Researchers have found that the doses listed on melatonin products may be very different from the amounts actually contained in the supplements. Choose only national, reputable brands or seek the advice of your healthcare professional.

? Did you know?

Melatonin first became available in 1993 in the United States as a dietary supplement. It was originally marketed as a cure for insomnia and jet lag.

PABA

WHAT IS IT?

PABA is the abbreviation for para-aminobenzoic acid, a compound that is an essential nutrient for microorganisms and some animals, but has not yet been shown to be essential for people. PABA is loosely considered by some to be a member of the vitamin B complex, though its actions differ widely from other B vitamins. PABA is best known for its work as a sunscreen. It helps block out skin-damaging ultraviolet rays. It's also an ingredient used by your body to make the vitamin folic acid. Oral PABA supplements won't help you make more folic acid though; only plants and certain bacteria can do that.

WHERE IS IT FOUND?

Most grains and animal foods contain PABA.

COMMON DOSES

The amount of PABA used for the conditions described above ranges from 300 mg per day, and up to 12 grams per day for autoimmune, connective tissue or skin disorders. Anyone taking more than 400 mg of PABA per day should consult a physician.

CLASSIFYING THE CLAIMS

Sound Science	Conflicting Science	Junk Science
	Enhances the effects of cortisone	Changes gray hair back to normal color Treats female infertility

! Think twice!

If you do take PABA supplements and sulfa antibiotics at the same time, PABA can cancel the antibiotic's effectiveness. Large amounts (8 grams per day or more) may cause low blood sugar, skin rash, fever and liver damage.

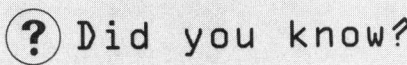

? Did you know?

PABA supplements won't make you sun-safe from the inside out.

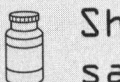

Shopping savvy

Small amounts of PABA are present in some B complex vitamins and multivitamin formulas.

Proanthocyanidins

WHAT ARE THEY?

Proanthocyanidins—also called "OPCs" for oligomeric proanthocyanidins or "PCOs" for pro-cyanidolic oligomers—are a class of nutrients belonging to the flavonoid family. Some researchers also call these molecules pycnogenol. The main functions of proanthocyanidins are antioxidant activity, and the stabilization of collagen and maintenance of elastin—two critical proteins in the connective tissue that supports organs and joints, as well as blood vessels and muscle.

WHERE ARE THEY FOUND?

Proanthocyanidins can be found in many plants, most notably pine bark, grape seed and grape skin.

However, bilberry, cranberry, black currant, green tea, black tea and other plants also contain these flavonoids. Nutritional supplements containing extracts of proanthocyanidins from various plant sources are available, alone or in combination with other nutrients, in herbal extracts, capsules and tablets.

COMMON DOSES

No safe or effective dose has been recommended. The manufacturers usually suggest proanthocyanidins at 50 to 100 mg per day.

CLASSIFYING THE CLAIMS		
Sound Science	**Conflicting Science**	**Junk Science**
Treats chronic venous insufficiency		Slows aging Treats AIDS Treats Alzheimer's disease Treats arthritis

! Think twice!

Proanthocyanidins have not been associated with any consistent side effects. As they are water-soluble nutrients, excess intake is probably excreted in the urine. However, no long-term studies have been completed that ensure safety over time.

? Did you know?

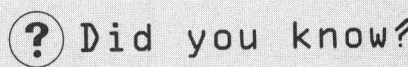

Pine tree bark extract is the source of pycnogenol.

Shopping savvy

Pine tree bark and grape seed extract are the main commercial sources of proanthocyanidins on the market. They can be used interchangeably, but most grape seed extract contains 92 to 95 percent proanthocyanidins, while pine tree bark extracts usually contain from 80 to 85 percent.

Probiotics

WHAT ARE THEY?

All bacteria aren't bad. Beneficial bacteria, such as *Lactobacillus acidophilus* and *Bifidobacterium bifidum*, are called probiotics. Probiotic bacteria favorably alter the intestinal microflora balance, inhibit the growth of harmful bacteria, promote good digestion, boost immune function and increase resistance to infection. Probiotic bacteria also produce substances called *bacteriocins*, which act as natural antibiotics to kill undesirable microorganisms. Individuals with flourishing intestinal colonies of beneficial bacteria are better equipped to fight the growth of disease-causing bacteria.

WHERE ARE THEY FOUND?

Beneficial bacteria present in fermented dairy foods—namely live culture yogurt—have been used as a folk remedy for hundreds, if not thousands, of years. Yogurt is the traditional source of beneficial bacteria; however, different brands of yogurt can vary greatly in their bacteria strain and potency. Some (particularly frozen) yogurts do not contain any live bacteria. Supplements in powder, liquid extract, capsule or tablet form containing beneficial bacteria are other sources of probiotics.

COMMON DOSES

The amount of probiotics necessary to replenish the intestines varies according to the extent of microbial depletion and the presence of harmful bacteria. One to two billion colony-forming units (CFUs) per day of acidophilus are considered to be the minimum beneficial amount for the healthy maintenance of intestinal microflora.

CLASSIFYING THE CLAIMS

Sound Science	Conflicting Science	Junk Science
Treats diarrhea	Treats canker sores	Treats cystic fibrosis
Prevents yeast infection	Enhances immune function	Treats indigestion

Individuals with compromised immune systems may be at increased risk for fungal infection from probiotics.

Certain medications may interact with probiotics.

Shopping savvy

Choose supplements containing bacteria that have been shown to have positive results. In addition to *Lactobacillus GG*, these include *Lactobacillus johnsoni*, *Lactobacillus reuteri*, and *Bifidobacterium*. *Lactobacillus GG* is one of a handful of probiotic bacteria strains available over the counter in capsule form.

Most commercial yogurt is pasteurized, a process that kills bacteria. Check the label for statements about the type and amount of cultures included.

? Did you know?

The digestive tract is home to more than 400 species of bacteria. Researchers believe that at least some of these native bugs crowd out invading organisms that cause illness by using resources that the bad bugs need and producing chemicals that kill them. Eat more of the helpful bacteria, the theory goes, and you can stave off stomach problems.

Diarrhea flushes intestinal microorganisms out of the gastrointestinal tract, leaving the body vulnerable to opportunistic infections. Replenishing the beneficial bacteria with probiotic supplements can help prevent new infections.

Psyllium

WHAT IS IT?

Psyllium is a bulk-forming laxative and is high in both fiber and mucilage. The laxative properties of psyllium are due to the swelling of the seeds or husks when they come in contact with water. A gelatinous mass then forms that help keeps feces hydrated and soft.

WHERE IS IT FOUND?

Psyllium is native to Iran and India and is currently cultivated in those countries. The seeds and husks are commonly used. Some grain products may have psyllium added as an ingredient to boost fiber or make a health claim—check the ingredient list.

COMMON DOSES

The suggested daily intake of psyllium husks is 4 to 20 grams (1 teaspoon) or 10 to 20 grams (up to 2 teaspoons) of the powdered seeds. This is stirred into a large glass of water or juice and drunk immediately before it thickens.

CLASSIFYING THE CLAIMS

Sound Science	Conflicting Science	Junk Science
Treats constipation	Aids weight loss	Treats psoriasis
Treats hemorrhoids	Lowers high triglycerides	Treats poison ivy and insect bites
Treats diabetes	Treats diarrhea	
Lowers high cholesterol		
Aids diverticulosis and irritable bowel syndrome		

! Think twice!

Diabetics who have difficulty regulating their blood sugar levels should not use psyllium.

Some allergic skin reactions and trouble breathing have been reported as side effects.

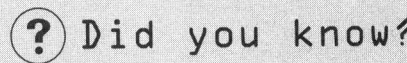 Did you know?

Psyllium powder is about half soluble fiber. If you take a 10-gram spoonful of powder, you will get about 5 grams of this beneficial fiber. Psyllium also comes in capsules and wafers and might be added to some fortified cereal products.

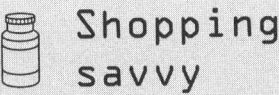 Shopping savvy

It is important to maintain a high water intake when using psyllium.

Quercetin

WHAT IS IT?

Quercetin belongs to a class of water-soluble plant pigments called flavonoids. Quercetin is also considered a phytoestrogen (plant substance with structural similarities to estrogen). Quercetin acts as an antihistamine and has anti-inflammatory properties. As an antioxidant, it protects LDL cholesterol (the "bad" cholesterol) from becoming damaged.

WHERE IS IT FOUND?

Quercetin can be found in red wine, purple grape juice, onions, apples, cranberries, green tea and black tea. Smaller amounts are found in leafy green vegetables and beans.

COMMON DOSES

Common supplemental intake of quercetin is 400 mg, 2 to 3 times per day.

CLASSIFYING THE CLAIMS		
Sound Science	Conflicting Science	Junk Science
Strengthens capillaries		Treats asthma
		Prevents cataracts
		Treats diabetes
		Lowers high cholesterol

⚠ Think twice!

Quercetin may increase the effects of adriamycin and cisplatin, two chemotherapy medications. More research is needed to determine whether quercetin should be taken in conjunction with chemotherapy.

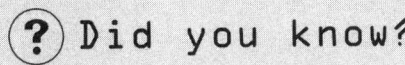

❓ Did you know?

There are more than 500 plants in the allium (or onion/lily) family. Red onions, yellow onions and shallots contain the highest natural levels of quercetin. You'll absorb more quercetin if you cook your onions instead of eating them raw.

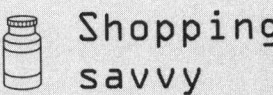

Shopping savvy

Since flavonoids help protect vitamin C, quercetin is often found in combination with vitamin C.

Royal Jelly

WHAT IS IT?

The thick, milky substance that is secreted from the glands of a special group of young nurse bees between their sixth and twelfth days of life is called royal jelly. When honey and pollen are combined and refined within the young nurse bee, royal jelly is born. Royal jelly is only made for the queen bee. It has no proven benefit for humans—even those with royal bloodlines.

WHERE IS IT FOUND?

Royal jelly is found only in beehives and supplements.

COMMON DOSAGE

No safe dose has been established. Manufacturers typically recommend 30 to 150 mg per day.

CLASSIFYING THE CLAIMS

Sound Science	Conflicting Science	Junk Science
	Potential antibiotic properties	Fights infection
		Slows aging
		Improves alertness
		Increases energy
		Reduces allergies and asthma

! Think twice!

Anyone allergic to bee stings should never take royal jelly or any product derived from bees.

Those with asthma may react to royal jelly or bee products with an attack.

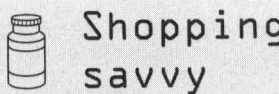

Shopping savvy

There is little, if any, good science to support claims for royal jelly, and no nutritional benefit to these supplements. Save your money.

? Did you know?

Only one bee per hive—the queen bee—eats royal jelly. The special nurse bees make royal jelly in the salivary glands. This saliva or spit is the main food source for the queen. It's a concentrated protein and mineral food—for the queen. Amounts of nutrients are so small they are insignificant to humans.

SAM-e

WHAT IS IT?

SAM-e (S-adenosyl-L-methionine, S-adenosylme-thionine) is an important biological agent in the human body required for more than 40 essential biochemical reactions. SAM-e participates in detoxi-fication reactions and in the manufacture of brain chemicals, antioxidants, joint tissue structures and many other important components. SAM-e is nor-mally produced in the liver from the amino acid methionine, which is abundant in most diets. Folic acid and vitamin B12 are necessary for the synthesis of SAM-e, and deficiencies of these vitamins result in low concentrations of SAM-e in your central nervous system.

WHERE IS IT FOUND?

SAM-e is not abundant in foods, but its amino acid precursor, methionine, is plentiful in most protein foods.

COMMON DOSES

SAM-e is commonly available in 100 and 200 mg tablets. No safe or recommended dose has been established. Clinical trials working with people suf-fering from a variety of conditions have been using these amounts of SAM-e: depression, 1,600 mg per day; osteoarthritis, 800 to 1,200 mg per day; fibromyalgia, 800 mg per day; liver disorders, 1,200 mg per day; and migraine, 800 mg per day.

CLASSIFYING THE CLAIMS

Sound Science	Conflicting Science	Junk Science
Treats cirrhosis of the liver Treats osteoarthritis	Treats depression	Treats fibromyalgia Treats migraine headaches

! Think twice!

Occasional gastrointestinal upset may be experienced.

Researchers treating people with bipolar disorder (manic depression) have reported that SAM-e could cause them to switch from depression to a manic episode. It is also not recommended for those with obsessive-compulsive disorder or addictive tendencies.

Use of SAM-e may be detrimental in people with Parkinson's disease. It can cause the depletion of dopamine and block the effects of L-dopa medications.

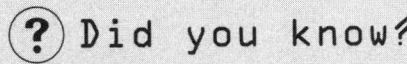

? Did you know?

SAM-e has been used for two decades in Europe to treat arthritis and depression, and is available only with a prescription. It first was discovered in the 1950s at the National Institutes of Health. In the 1970s, an Italian lab learned to produce it in cell cultures, and studied its use as an antidepressant. Some of the first patients who were given SAM-e for depression also suffered with osteoarthritis. The antiarthritic potential of SAM-e was realized when some people reported relief from their joint pain as well as their depression.

Shopping savvy

Supplements of SAM-e have been available in the United States just since 1997. Choose SAM-e supplements that contain butanedisulfonate—the newest, most stable form of this product.

Shark Cartilage

WHAT IS IT?

Shark cartilage supplements became popular among cancer patients based on the theory that if sharks rarely get cancer, there must be something in them that could solve the cancer mystery in humans. Scientists have found that certain compounds in shark cartilage have "anti-angiogenic" properties, which means they block the growth of the tiny blood vessels that feed tumors. As a result of studies on shark cartilage, two new anti-angiogenic drugs, angiostatin and endostatin, are currently being investigated. However, no studies have been completed to date.

WHERE IS IT FOUND?

Shark cartilage is taken from the dorsal fins of shark. This supplement has become so popular and lucrative that some companies harvest live shark from the ocean, cut off their fins and toss them back into the ocean to die.

COMMON DOSES

There are no safe or recommended doses for shark cartilage. Manufacturers' labels suggest 15 to 20 gram doses, 3 to 4 times a day.

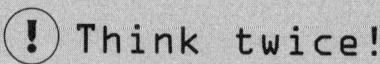

Side effects may include nausea, vomiting and constipation. There has been one reported case of hepatitis associated with supplementation of shark cartilage.

CLASSIFYING THE CLAIMS

Sound Science	Conflicting Science	Junk Science
Anti-angiogenic properties		Cures cancer

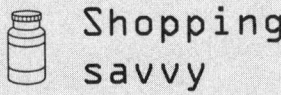
Shopping savvy

With a cost of up to $1,000 a month, terminally ill patients might find a better use for their money.

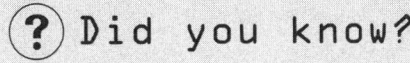
Did you know?

Shark cartilage promoters say it takes 16 to 20 weeks for the cancer-fighting agents to work. Four or five months is a long time for someone with cancer to try an alternative therapy.

Soy Isoflavones

WHAT ARE THEY?

Soybeans contain a unique group of phytochemicals called isoflavones, which are also known as phyto-estrogens. Soy products are the only food that contains genistein. This compound helps stop the growth of tumors and can lower cholesterol in those with high levels in their blood. Soy protein differs from other vegetable proteins because it changes how the liver processes cholesterol. To gain heart health benefits, you have to eat at least 25 grams of soy protein a day to consume enough isoflavones to make a health difference.

WHERE ARE THEY FOUND?

Soybeans are the only source of soy isoflavones. Soybeans are one of the major sources of protein worldwide. Soy may be added to many different types of foods and beverages. It is used to make tofu, some types of noodles, and meat substitutes such as soy burgers. Soymilk is frequently prescribed for babies allergic to other types of milk.

COMMON DOSES

Most researchers agree that you need at least 25 grams of soy protein per day to gain beneficial effects.

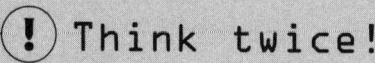

(!) Think twice!

The weak estrogen-like activity of soy isoflavones may stimulate the growth of some cancer cells.

CLASSIFYING THE CLAIMS

Sound Science	Conflicting Science	Junk Science
Reduces risk for heart disease as part of an overall low-fat diet	Natural substitute for hormone replacement therapy (HRT)	

Shopping savvy

The FDA has approved a food label claim for foods that contain at least 6.25 grams of soy protein per serving. Research has shown that 25 grams of soy protein daily, as part of a diet low in fat and cholesterol, may reduce the risk of heart disease. Check the food label to determine the amount of soy present.

Did you know?

Soy foods that undergo certain types of processing have few, if any, soy isoflavones remaining. Using lots of water, alcohol or repeated washings during processing removes this key ingredient. Common foods that are low in soy isoflavones include textured soy protein, soymilk and soy oil.

Spirulina

WHAT IS IT?

Spirulina is a form of freshwater blue-green algae rich in chlorophyll just like all green or blue-green foods. Also known as blue-green algae, this single-celled microorganism resembles bacteria. It contains small amounts of B-complex vitamins, beta-carotene, iron and protein. Spirulina is used in animal feed, as a coloring agent and in supplements.

WHERE IS IT FOUND?

Spirulina grows naturally in Mexico and certain parts of Africa. Currently, spirulina is marketed in tablets, capsules, powders and as an ingredient in smoothies, snack foods and energy bars.

COMMON DOSES

No safe dosage has been established. Manufacturers typically recommend 3 to 20 grams per day.

CLASSIFYING THE CLAIMS		
Sound Science	**Conflicting Science**	**Junk Science**
	Treats severe malnutrition	Treats diabetes
		Treats hypoglycemia
		Treats drug addiction
		Treats alcoholism

! Think twice!

Anyone with a compromised immune system should avoid spirulina. The potential contamination with germs and bacteria could be deadly.

"Cleansing" reactions such as headaches, tiredness, runny nose, constipation or diarrhea may appear. Other symptoms, such as fatigue, skin rashes, nervousness and increased susceptibility to colds will supposedly pass after about a week, tout manufacturers. Often, people are told not to use any medication that suppresses these symptoms and to avoid high-protein foods because it can compromise the healing process. This is not good advice.

Individuals on blood thinning medications (like Coumadin) should avoid spirulina, because it may increase their risk for blood clots and stroke.

? Did you know?

The original source of spirulina was pond scum (algae) from Lake Texcoco, a polluted lake outside of Mexico City. Most of the algae used in spirulina are now cultivated in clean ponds.

Shopping savvy

Spirulina is expensive, tastes terrible and doesn't provide high levels of any nutrient. Save your money.

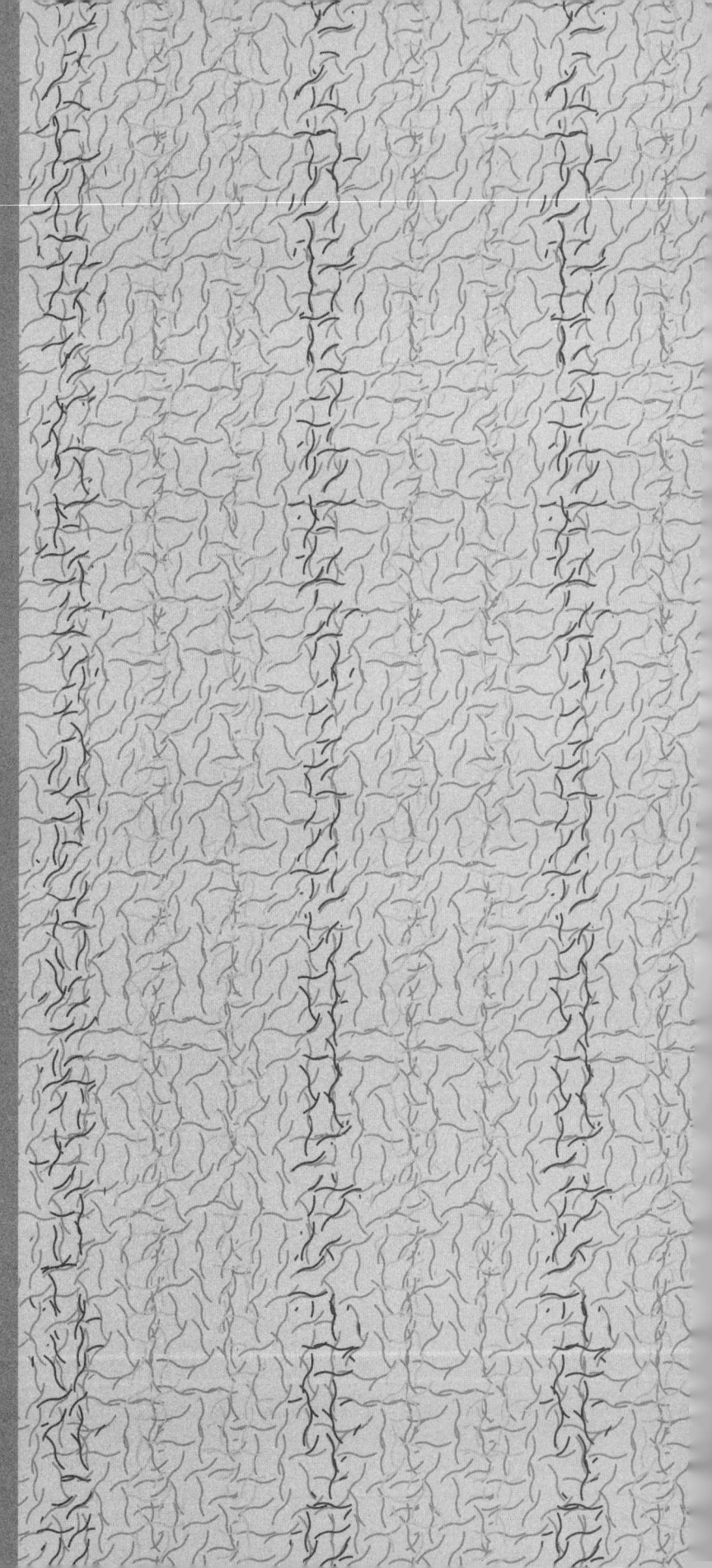

Conditions

If you have a specific condition or ailment (or are concerned about one), you should never just sit back and suffer (or worry). Working with healthcare professionals is of course your first course of action. But there are also ways that nutrition—vitamins, minerals and supplements—might be able to solve the challenges you're up against. In fact, sometimes the solutions are downright simple.

How to Use This Chapter

*This chapter details the most common conditions that may benefit from
nutrition therapy. Each condition is described from a variety of angles:*

Common Symptoms
Common symptoms are
listed to help you identify
early signs of the condition.

Overview
A discussion of the condition,
its forms, and its prevalence.

What Is It?
Provides a brief, understandable summary of the disease
or ailment.

Who's At Risk?
Provides categories of people
who are most likely to be
affected.

CONDITIONS

236

Smart Nutrition

Arthritis, Rheumatoid

Rheumatoid arthritis is not just a benign
process that causes the joints to hurt. It's a
disease that causes a fair amount of damage
to joints, and it can start causing that damage within
the first couple of years. In this less common but
more debilitating form of arthritis, the immune system attacks healthy joints, causing inflammation,
pain and sometimes disfiguring joint damage.

The cause of rheumatoid arthritis is unknown.
Rheumatoid arthritis is linked to overall poor nutritional status. The inflammatory process of arthritis
changes your intestinal lining and reduces the
absorption of some nutrients. Often, the long-term
medications used to treat chronic pain and swelling
can increase nutrient needs beyond normal
requirements.

WHAT IS IT?

Rheumatoid arthritis is a disease that affects the
joints. It's an inflammatory disease as opposed to the
wear-and-tear type of destruction that typifies
osteo-arthritis. Rheumatoid arthritis causes joints to
swell and to become stiff and sore. The immune system attacks joints and other tissues as if they were
foreign invaders. Actually, an inflammatory response
is quite normal. For example, if you cut yourself
you will notice that there will be some redness and
swelling in the area; that's a normal part of the healing response. But in people who have rheumatoid
arthritis, something has gone wrong and that inflammatory response starts for unknown reasons, then
continues and doesn't stop. Instead of the inflammatory response helping to heal, it causes harm.

▶ **Common symptoms**

- Soreness
- Stiffness and aching in muscles and
  joints
- Pain and swelling in joints
- Loss of motion of the affected joints
- Loss of strength in muscles attached to
  the affected joints
- Fatigue, which can be severe during a
  flare-up
- Low-grade fever
- Deformity of the joints over time

☞ **Who's at risk?**

- Those with a family history
- Possibly individuals exposed to certain
  viruses

Nutrition Recommendations
Nutrition recommendations include strategies for eating to protect your health and ward off or delay the onset of disease. Suggestions include cooking tips, menu planning ideas and strategies for caregivers.

Did You Know?
Common questions or concerns are addressed here to help you separate fact from fiction.

NUTRITION RECOMMENDATIONS

Maintain a healthy weight.
Eat more fish meals—at least 3 or 4 a week—for omega-3 fatty acids.
Aim for 25 to 35 grams of fiber daily from fruits, vegetables, whole grains and legumes.
Choose breads and cereals with flaxseed.
Make use of energy-saving devices and easy-open containers to help save wear on your joints.
Add fresh peppers, grated carrots, mushrooms and onions canned or jarred spaghetti sauce to boost fiber and nutrients.
Add extra vegetables to rice mixes.
Buy ready-to-eat leafy salad greens.
Cook and serve in the same dish whenever possible to save on clean up and moving of dishes.

❓ Did you know?

Biologic agents are a promising new treatment for those who suffer with rheumatoid arthritis. Tumor necrosis factor (TNF) is a naturally occurring protein produced in high quantities by cells that are involved in inflammation. TNF causes the symptoms that occur with rheumatoid arthritis, such as pain and swelling, but also produces agents that damage the joint itself. New drugs are being tested that can bind and clear away TNF. This new category of drugs won't cure your arthritis, but it might improve how you feel and can potentially reduce joint injury which would otherwise occur.

237

SUPPLEMENT SUGGESTIONS

▶ A multivitamin/mineral supplement with 100 to 150 percent of the RDA is recommended for those with rheumatoid arthritis.
▶ Consider taking 1 tablespoon of flaxseed or flaxseed oil daily.
▶ If you can't or won't eat more fish, consider a fish oil supplement.
▶ If you take the medication methotrexate, an anti-folate agent for rheumatoid arthritis, ask your physician about whether to supplement with folic acid.

🗎 Startling statistics

Rheumatoid arthritis affects about 2.5 million Americans. It's three times more common in women than in men and generally strikes between the ages of 20 and 50, but it also can affect very young children and adults over age 50.

Startling Statistics
These will help you put things into perspective.

Supplement Suggestions
Here you'll find the most current, scientific recommendations for increased or decreased nutrient needs.

Alcoholism

You probably know someone who abuses alcohol. It's a fairly common problem, affecting about 10 percent of the population in the United States. Alcohol hinders your ability to absorb, process, use and store nutrients. Just as damaging is that alcohol intake at high levels pushes out other foods you might have eaten. If you drink a lot, you're consuming empty calories. Alcohol has toxic effects on the whole gastrointestinal tract and cripples the ability to remove and use nutrients from the foods you eat. Long-term alcohol abuse usually leads to liver damage, which significantly reduces your ability to store and use most nutrients.

WHAT IS IT?

Moderate drinking is defined as 1 or fewer drinks per day for women and 2 or fewer drinks per day for men. And no, you can't save them up from day to day! Excessive drinking—more than 3 drinks per day for women and 6 for men—increases risk of cancer and can damage the liver, intestines, pancreas and brain. It can cause diarrhea, osteoporosis, night blindness and anemia and can take about 15 years from your life span.

▶ Common symptoms

- Confusion
- Poor coordination
- Poor memory
- Underweight
- Unsteady gait

Who's at risk?

- Those with a family history of alcoholism

NUTRITION RECOMMENDATIONS

The best nutritional advice is to abstain from alcohol; it is toxic to your body and interferes with absorption of most nutrients.

✔ Eat a variety of foods, especially fruits, vegetables and whole grains.

✔ Try eating smaller, more frequent meals if you can't manage larger portions.

✔ Drink plenty of water to stay hydrated, as alcohol has a dehydrating effect.

✔ Limit coffee and tea consumption, both decaf and regular, as they compound nutrient absorption problems.

SUPPLEMENT SUGGESTIONS

▶ Individuals with a large alcohol intake should take a multivitamin/mineral supplement with 100 to 150 percent of the RDA.

▶ Men should not exceed 5,000 IU of vitamin A; women should not exceed 4,000 IU of vitamin A—such doses of vitamin A can be toxic to your liver when combined with heavy alcohol use.

▶ Vitamin, mineral or nutritional supplements cannot treat or cure an alcohol addiction.

(?) Did you know?

A thiamin deficiency from alcohol abuse damages brain cells that may lead to Wernicke-Korsakoff syndrome, a brain disorder characterized by unsteady gait and memory loss.

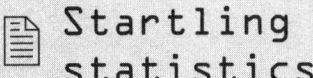

Startling statistics

About 50 percent of fatal car accidents involve a drinking driver.

Allergies, Food

In homes, schools and institutions around the country, people are eliminating certain foods from their diets, believing that allergic reactions to those foods are causing physical and emotional problems. Because you eat a variety of foods daily, it's easy to associate an unexplained symptom or discomfort with food. When you eliminate any food, you could be limiting your access to important vitamins and minerals. Many people claim to be allergic to a food. But a true allergy is quite different from a food intolerance or sensitivity, which is what most people really have. The symptoms are similar, but these reactions—unlike allergies—either don't involve the immune system, or they involve a different part of the immune system than true allergies do.

WHAT IS IT?

An allergic reaction occurs when your immune system mistakes a particular food as a harmful invader. Histamine and other chemicals are launched to attack the food in a misguided effort to protect you from harm. This is the same system that responds to insect stings. Allergic reactions are also called anaphylaxis and can sometimes lead to death if not promptly treated.

ALLERGIC OR NOT?

To help distinguish between foods you just don't like, a food intolerance, and a true food allergy, ask yourself the following questions:

* *After eating certain foods, do you break out into a rash, have itching, swelling, gastrointestinal problems, or trouble breathing?*

* *Do symptoms appear within minutes or up to two hours after eating the food?*

* *Do you have a history of asthma or allergies to other things?*
* *Do allergies run in your family?*

If you answered "yes" to most of these questions, then food allergy is more likely, as opposed to food intolerance. If you know that every time you eat a certain food you have a reaction, then it makes sense to avoid that food. If you aren't sure of the offending food, try an elimination diet under a doctor's or dietitian's supervision.

▶ Common symptoms

- Hives
- Swelling (especially of the lips and face)
- Difficulty breathing (because of swelling in the throat or an asthmatic reaction)
- Vomiting
- Diarrhea
- Cramping
- Sudden drop in blood pressure

Anaphylaxis can be sudden or appear more like a slowly developing illness, making it the most dangerous reaction. Some noted allergists believe that repeated exposure to certain medicines or food ingredients can weaken the lining of your intestines. That makes it easier for allergens to pass through this barrier and come in direct contact with your immune system, provoking a reaction.

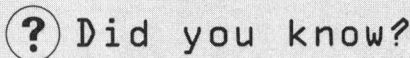

☞ Who's at risk?

- Individuals with a family or personal history of food or other allergies

NUTRITION RECOMMENDATIONS

Before you eliminate foods from your diet, check with a board-certified allergist to determine if you have a true allergy. Immune therapy or allergy shots have not been proven to really work, nor has oral desensitization helped in eliminating food allergies. Bottom line: If you have a true food allergy, avoid the food.

✔ *Eat more fruits, vegetables and whole grains that are rich in antioxidants that help keep your immune system strong.*

✔ *At restaurants, always identify that you have a food allergy. Ask how a food was prepared and see that your waitperson checks with the chef to determine if any of the offending food is included in your selection. Never taste foods before asking questions.*

✔ *At the supermarket, read food ingredient lists carefully. Become familiar with unfamiliar names used on labels; for example, sodium caseinate and casein are ingredients to avoid if you are allergic to milk protein. If you have questions about favorite foods, contact the manufacturers of the product.*

SUPPLEMENT SUGGESTIONS

▶ A multivitamin/mineral supplement is recommended for those with food allergies. Additional supplements may be needed if you have a large number of allergies or are allergic to milk products. Check with your healthcare provider for specific recommendations.

▶ Be sure to check the ingredient label of your supplements to be sure they do not contain potential allergens.

? Did you know?

Milk, eggs, shellfish (especially shrimp), soy, fish, wheat, legumes, peanuts and tree nuts (such as walnuts), frequently contain allergens. Childhood allergies to egg, milk, soy or wheat are often outgrown. Allergies developed as an adult are typically with you for life.

If you have a severe allergy, always carry self-injectable epinephrine, and use it at the first hint of a strong reaction. Ask your doctor for a prescription.

229

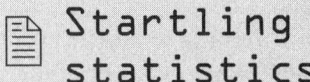

📄 Startling statistics

About 150 people a year in the United States die from anaphylactic shock caused by a food allergy.

Alzheimer's Disease

About 4 million Americans have Alzheimer's disease, which each year claims 100,000 lives in the United States. Worldwide, experts estimate that 5 percent of people over 65, and up to 40 percent of those over 80, have Alzheimer's disease, an eventually fatal deterioration of mental function. Alzheimer's disease is the most common form of dementia.

There have been some important advances in Alzheimer's disease research. Scientists discovered a previously unknown abnormal change in the brains of patients with Alzheimer's disease, called the AMY plaque. This new discovery may lead researchers to a better understanding of the disease and to the development of new therapies. Ongoing studies of the inflammatory processes of the brain point to the potential beneficial use of anti-inflammatory medication in treating or slowing the progression of the disease.

WHAT IS IT?

People with Alzheimer's have characteristic brain features that were first noted by Alois Alzheimer in 1907. These unusual features include brain atrophy (shrinkage), the accumulation of plaques and tangles in the brain, and the degeneration of neurons. There are also excess amounts of other nutrients like calcium, silicon, sulfur and bromine, and deficiencies of potassium, selenium, vitamin B12 and zinc. It's not known whether high levels of any nutrients are a cause or a result of Alzheimer's. We still don't know what causes Alzheimer's, and no effective treatment exists to stop this disease. Because clinical tests for Alzheimer's are often inconclusive, brain dissection at autopsy is still the only way to confirm this diagnosis.

High levels of the amino acid homocysteine (already linked to increased risk of heart disease) are also associated with Alzheimer's disease. In heart disease, the higher the level of homocysteine in the blood, the greater the risk of damage to the artery lining. That, in turn, leads to the buildup of plaque in the artery wall. In Alzheimer's, homocysteine may similarly damage the vessel linings—but, in this case, the lining of small blood vessels in the brain is affected. This, in turn, decreases blood flow to certain brain areas, and may predispose some people to the brain plaques that characterize Alzheimer's.

▶ Common symptoms

There are 3 progressive stages of Alzheimer's disease:

AMNESIA STAGE
- Trouble with short-term memory
- Tend to ask the same questions over and over
- Forget telephone numbers
- Have trouble with math and visual-motor skills

CONFUSION STAGE
- Impaired reading and writing
- Failure to identify common objects and sounds
- Disorientation of time and place
- Personality change
- Extreme aggressiveness and wandering

DEMENTIA STAGE
- Completely withdrawn and unresponsive
- Bedridden

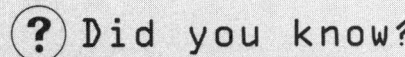

Who's at risk?

- Older women not on hormone replacement therapy
- Those with a family history of Alzheimer's
- People with a history of head trauma

NUTRITION RECOMMENDATIONS

People with Alzheimer's need optimal nutrition and often are not capable of managing this on their own. Caregivers should carefully monitor meal planning and eating.

✔ *Eat plenty of fruits and vegetables. A well-balanced diet with at least five servings of fresh fruits and vegetables per day is the best way to keep homocysteine levels normal, experts say. Dark green leafy vegetables, orange juice and organ meats are also good sources of folic acid.*

✔ *Choose fortified whole grains. Since fortification of enriched cereal grains began, folic acid can be found in enriched bread, pasta, flour, cereal, rice and many other foods in the United States.*

✔ *Smaller, more frequent meals can help increase food intake since appetite is often diminished.*

✔ *Finger foods are more manageable for those in the advanced stages of the disease. Making foods easy to eat will help boost nutrition intake.*

✔ *Limit caffeine intake. Drinking five or more cups of coffee a day raises homocysteine levels.*

✔ *Engage in a more active lifestyle. Walk instead of drive, and take the stairs instead of the elevator. Sedentary lifestyles have been linked to Alzheimer's disease.*

SUPPLEMENT SUGGESTIONS

▶ A multivitamin/mineral supplement providing RDAs of 100 to 150 percent is recommended for those with Alzheimer's disease.

▶ It may be possible to delay some cases of Alzheimer's disease through supplementation with folic acid and other B vitamins. Folic acid and B vitamins break down homocysteine in the body, thereby reducing blood levels.

? Did you know?

Alzheimer's is not a normal part of the aging process.

Well-nourished people fight off disease more easily and help stabilize mental capability, daily function and alertness. Many people with Alzheimer's consume very low levels of vitamins and minerals, particularly vitamin A, several of the B vitamins, calcium, iron and zinc. These substances are essential for body and brain health.

Startling statistics

It's estimated that half of all women over 80 will develop some form of dementia that shows up as a significant decline in intelligence and social skills.

The brain contains as many as 100 billion cells that make up a complex communication relay system and control center for body operations.

Anemia, Iron Deficiency

The most common type of anemia is iron deficiency anemia. Women of childbearing age and young children are most susceptible to iron deficiency anemia. It takes a long time for this type of anemia to occur. Infants whose mothers had poor iron status during pregnancy are likely to be anemic, as are babies not breast-fed or given infant formula that is not iron-fortified. Before menopause, women need almost twice as much iron as men do, because of the menstrual blood they lose each month.

WHAT IS IT?

"Iron poor, tired blood" is a good way to describe anemia. It's a blood condition in which the number and/or size of the red blood cells are reduced. Because red blood cells move oxygen from your lungs to the tissues, any decrease in size or amount limits how much oxygen is transported.

☛ Who's at risk?

- Infants
- Teenage girls
- Menstruating women with heavy monthly blood losses
- Pregnant women
- Accident victims with significant blood losses
- People on low-calorie diets
- Alcoholics
- People with gastrointestinal ulcers or other internal bleeding

NUTRITION RECOMMENDATIONS

It's not that there aren't enough iron-rich foods; there are plenty. The problem is that there are many obstacles to absorbing the iron from foods. There are two forms of iron: heme and nonheme. Heme iron (found in meat) is absorbed at a rate of 30 to 40 percent. Compare that to nonheme iron (from plants), only 3 to 4 percent of the available iron is absorbed. About 40 percent of the iron in meat foods are heme iron, but all the iron in plant foods is nonheme.

✔ *Choose a healthful variety of foods, especially those rich in iron such as lean red meat.*

✔ *Include plenty of foods rich in vitamin C when you do*

▶ Common symptoms

- ■ Fatigue
- ■ Weakness
- ■ Pale skin
- ■ Shortness of breath
- ■ Palpitations
- ■ Heart failure
- ■ Shock

eat foods that contain iron. The vitamin C will help absorb more of the available iron from foods or supplements.

✔ *Use cast-iron cookware. Tiny iron particles from the cookware are transferred to food and can provide a significant source of dietary iron.*

SUPPLEMENT SUGGESTIONS

▸ Keep all iron supplements in a locked cabinet, out of the reach of children. Accidental iron overdose is the number one cause of fatal poisoning in young children.

? Did you know?

Eating just a little bit of meat can significantly improve the absorption of all iron in a meal. "Meat factor" is the name of the substance believed to cause this effect. If you can't or won't eat meat, then the acidity from foods that contain vitamin C (ascorbic acid) can boost nonheme iron absorption.

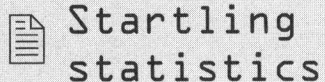

Startling statistics

On average, only about 10 percent of the iron you eat is absorbed. Your body is incredibly adept at hoarding iron. The less you eat, the more you absorb. That's why vegetarians do not have higher rates of anemia than meat eaters. However, this adaptation only goes so far. If you get far too little iron, you can't catch up.

Arthritis, Osteo

rthritis is the common name for more than 100 different rheumatic diseases, which result in pain, degeneration and inflammation of the joints. The single most significant nutrition tool in managing arthritis is maintaining a healthy weight. Symptoms of osteoarthritis often subside when excess pounds are shed.

WHAT IS IT?

Osteoarthritis, the most common form, results when the cartilage that cushions joint bones deteriorates. With age, the smooth linings of your joints begin to deteriorate and become roughened or cracked. The bone underneath these joints becomes thickened as a result. Osteoarthritis usually affects the larger joints such as hips and knees, but it can attack any joint in the body.

▶ Common symptoms

- ■ Joint pain
- ■ Joint stiffness
- ■ Joint swelling

☞ Who's at risk?

- • Overweight and obese individuals
- • Ballet dancers
- • Football players
- • Professional athletes
- • Individuals with repeated injury to the same joint
- • Anyone who's had a major trauma to a joint

NUTRITION RECOMMENDATIONS

Because arthritis symptoms come and go, it's tempting to blame foods for flare-ups. There is no evidence that any food triggers arthritis symptoms.

✔ *Maintain a healthy weight. If you have osteoarthritis of the knee, losing weight will reduce stress on your joints. Every additional pound of weight is equal to three pounds of pressure on your knees.*

✔ *Eat a generous variety of fruits and vegetables, whole grains, skim or low-fat dairy products, legumes and fish.*

✔ *Regular physical activity helps strengthen muscles, keeps joints flexible and aids mobility. Try activities that don't strain joints, like swimming or walking. Best of all, exercise can improve functioning without increasing symptoms. A lack of exercise, on the other hand, leads to weakening and breakdown of cartilage.*

✔ *Cayenne from hot peppers stimulates blood flow, loosening up any blockages associated with stiff, inflamed joints.*

✔ *Seek a doctor's advice. Getting prompt treatment can help slow or prevent damage that might otherwise progress. In order to prevent possible drug/nutrient interactions, be sure to tell the doctor which supplements you take.*

✔ *Overuse of non-steroidal anti-inflammatory drugs (NSAIDs), such as aspirin and ibuprofen, can cause severe complications like internal bleeding and liver and kidney damage.*

SUPPLEMENT SUGGESTIONS

▶ A multivitamin/mineral supplement with 100 to 150 percent of the RDA is recommend for those with osteoarthritis.

▶ Glucosamine may also be helpful. Most research suggests a dose of 500 mg of glucosamine hydrochloride or sulfate, three times a day.

? Did you know?

Almost everyone over age 40 shows some signs of osteoarthritis on x-rays, even if they have no symptoms. This type of arthritis is a consequence of aging and is not the same as rheumatoid arthritis.

A common diet remedy is avoiding the "nightshade" family of vegetables (eggplant, tomatoes, peppers and potatoes). There is no proof these foods have any effect on arthritis. However, it's easy to avoid particular foods if you think they are a problem. But beware: If you eliminate any category or group of foods from your diet, you risk nutritional deficiencies that, in turn, can aggravate your arthritis over the long run.

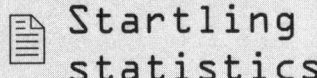

Startling statistics

Unfortunately, there is no cure for arthritis. It's not surprising, then, that arthritis ranks second only to cancer in the number of bogus "miracle cures." Americans spend about $1 billion a year on unproved arthritis remedies. Though there is growing evidence that some nutrition remedies may be helpful, no single therapy can be expected to work for every type of arthritis.

Forty million Americans have some form of arthritis. As the population ages, this number will increase to 60 million by the year 2020. That's one in every five people.

Arthritis, Rheumatoid

Rheumatoid arthritis is not just a benign process that causes the joints to hurt. It's a disease that causes a fair amount of damage to joints, and it can start causing that damage within the first couple of years. In this less common but more debilitating form of arthritis, the immune system attacks healthy joints, causing inflammation, pain and sometimes disfiguring joint damage.

The cause of rheumatoid arthritis is unknown. Rheumatoid arthritis is linked to overall poor nutritional status. The inflammatory process of arthritis changes your intestinal lining and reduces the absorption of some nutrients. Often, the long-term medications used to treat chronic pain and swelling can increase nutrient needs beyond normal requirements.

What Is It?

Rheumatoid arthritis is a disease that affects the joints. It's an inflammatory disease as opposed to the wear-and-tear type of destruction that typifies osteo-arthritis. Rheumatoid arthritis causes joints to swell and to become stiff and sore. The immune system attacks joints and other tissues as if they were foreign invaders. Actually, an inflammatory response is quite normal. For example, if you cut yourself you will notice that there will be some redness and swelling in the area; that's a normal part of the healing response. But in people who have rheumatoid arthritis, something has gone wrong and that inflammatory response starts for unknown reasons, then continues and doesn't stop. Instead of the inflammatory response helping to heal, it causes harm.

▶ **Common symptoms**

- Soreness
- Stiffness and aching in muscles and joints
- Pain and swelling in joints
- Loss of motion of the affected joints
- Loss of strength in muscles attached to the affected joints
- Fatigue, which can be severe during a flare-up
- Low-grade fever
- Deformity of the joints over time

☞ **Who's at risk?**

- Those with a family history
- Possibly individuals exposed to certain viruses

NUTRITION RECOMMENDATIONS

- ✔ *Maintain a healthy weight.*
- ✔ *Eat more fish meals—at least 3 or 4 a week—for omega-3 fatty acids.*
- ✔ *Aim for 25 to 35 grams of fiber daily from fruits, vegetables, whole grains and legumes.*
- ✔ *Choose breads and cereals with flaxseed.*
- ✔ *Make use of energy-saving devices and easy-open containers to help save wear on your joints.*
- ✔ *Add fresh peppers, grated carrots, mushrooms and onions to canned or jarred spaghetti sauce to boost fiber and nutrients.*
- ✔ *Add extra vegetables to rice mixes.*
- ✔ *Buy ready-to-eat leafy salad greens.*
- ✔ *Cook and serve in the same dish whenever possible to save on clean up and moving of dishes.*

SUPPLEMENT SUGGESTIONS

▸ A multivitamin/mineral supplement with 100 to 150 percent of the RDA is recommended for those with rheumatoid arthritis.

▸ Consider taking 1 tablespoon of flaxseed or flaxseed oil daily.

▸ If you can't or won't eat more fish, consider a fish oil supplement.

▸ If you take the medication methotrexate, an antifolate agent for rheumatoid arthritis, ask your physician about whether to supplement with folic acid.

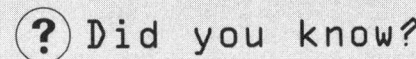

(?) Did you know?

Biologic agents are a promising new treatment for those who suffer with rheumatoid arthritis. Tumor necrosis factor (TNF) is a naturally occurring protein produced in high quantities by cells that are involved in inflammation. TNF causes the symptoms that occur with rheumatoid arthritis, such as pain and swelling, but also produces agents that damage the joint itself. New drugs are being tested that can bind and clear away TNF. This new category of drugs won't cure your arthritis, but it might improve how you feel and can potentially reduce joint injury which would otherwise occur.

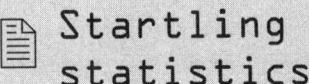

Startling statistics

Rheumatoid arthritis affects about 2.5 million Americans. It's three times more common in women than in men and generally strikes between the ages of 20 and 50, but it also can affect very young children and adults over age 50.

Asthma

A sthma has dramatically risen worldwide over the past decades, particularly in developed countries. Asthma has increased by 60 percent in the United States since the early 1980s, and in Europe it has doubled in the same time frame. Children under the age of 4 have had the most dramatic increase in this disease, and the experts are still trying to determine why. Asthma is most likely a result of genetic susceptibility, which probably involves several genes, and various triggers, such as infections, dietary patterns, hormonal changes in women, and allergens.

WHAT IS IT?

When air can't pass freely to and from the tiny air sacs in the lungs, bronchial asthma occurs. Spasms in the muscles surrounding the small branches of the lungs tighten. This constriction reduces the outward passage of stale air.

A person who has any type of allergy may be at increased risk for asthma. Some children with asthma, who are also allergic to at least one food, may fail to respond positively to asthma treatment unless they avoid the offending foods, especially eggs, wheat, cow's milk, soy and fish. Several sulfites in food products can also be a factor in asthma attacks. These can be found in preservatives for salads, dips, cut or sliced fruit, coleslaw, potato products and other prepared foods.

Vitamin B6 has been studied for its effect on reducing wheezing. People with asthma tend to have low blood levels of B6. Supplements usually don't work to raise blood levels, but they may decrease the severity, occurrence and length of an asthma attack.

The antioxidant nutrients, vitamins C, E, beta-carotene and selenium, may have a role in reducing the risk of asthma. It's interesting to note that blood levels of vitamin C temporarily drop during an asthma attack. There is no research to show why this happens or whether taking additional vitamin C may prevent or lessen the severity of the attack.

▶ Common symptoms

- Coughing
- Wheezing
- Tight chest
- Difficulty breathing

☞ Who's at risk?

- Those with a family history of allergies or asthma
- Heavy exposure to pollutants or irritants
- Exposure to cigarette smoke

NUTRITION RECOMMENDATIONS

✔ Maintain a healthy weight, especially in childhood.
✔ Eat more fruits, vegetables and whole grains rich in antioxidants to enhance your immune function.

SUPPLEMENT SUGGESTIONS

▸ Those with asthma should take a multivitamin/mineral supplement with 100 to 150 percent of the RDA.

▸ Consider 100 mg/day supplements of B6 for a short time (3 to 4 weeks) to determine if they might lessen the intensity of your attacks.

▸ Exercise-induced asthma may be avoided with supplements of vitamin C one hour prior to exercise. Check with your healthcare professional for specific dose recommendations.

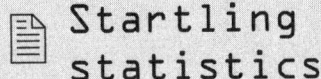
Startling statistics

More than 4,000 people die each year from serious asthma attacks.

Asthma is the third major cause of hospitalization in children under 15.

? Did you know?

The repeated inflammation that occurs with each episode of asthma can change the shape and function of an asthma sufferer's airways, a process known as remodeling. The airways become smaller, making it more difficult for air to pass freely. The exact causes of remodeling are not known, but current research suggests it may be a combination of overproduction of mucus, scarring, or the presence of specific white blood cells caused neutrophils. Over the course of many years, remodeling causes irreversible changes in the airways of a person with asthma, and may result in chronic asthma. The bottom line is that preventing asthmatic attacks can help decrease your risk for chronic asthma.

Cancer

In 1997, the World Cancer Research Fund and the American Institute for Cancer Research issued a comprehensive report on how we could slash cancer rates simply by changing what we eat and how much we exercise. Sometimes people think, "I've got the genes, I'll get the disease." We are now beginning to understand that cancer is preventable despite family histories, just as heart disease is. But cancer is a lot more complicated. Unlike heart disease, cancer is many unique diseases that attack different organs that have different risk factors.

One thing is absolutely clear: A diet high in fruits and vegetables is associated with a lower risk of cancer at almost every site on the body. This link with fruits and vegetables was not clear before the 1990s.

What Is It?

Cancer accounts for more than 100 different diseases, but all cancers have one thing in common. A cancer is the result of cells that lack controls to stop the growth process, so they continue to multiply without restraint. Cancer cells compete with healthy cells for both nutrients and space. These out-of-control cells may invade nearby structures and can sometimes break away and spread to distant parts of your body. Lung, breast, prostate and colon are the big four cancers for Americans. Smoking raises the rate of pancreatic cancer. Lymphoma and melanoma are both rising, but there's no evidence that diet is involved. Kidney cancer is also on the rise; it's associated with obesity.

▶ Common symptoms

- Change in bowel or bladder habits
- Sore that does not heal
- Unusual bleeding or discharge
- Thickening or lump in the breast or elsewhere
- Indigestion or difficulty swallowing
- Obvious change in a wart or mole
- Nagging cough or hoarseness

☞ Who's at risk?

- Smokers
- Those exposed to asbestos, arsenic and other chemicals
- Those overexposed to the sun
- Those with high-fat and/or low-fiber eating styles
- Those who overconsume alcohol

Nutrition Recommendations

No single food or nutrient causes or prevents cancer. Choose a low-fat eating plan that includes plenty of fruits, vegetables and whole grains. A high-fat diet is linked to breast, colon and prostate cancers.

✔ Trim all meat, poultry and fish of fatty deposits before

cooking. This will reduce your fat intake and decrease your exposure to harmful toxins that are stored in fatty tissue.

✔ Maintain a healthy weight, and get regular physical activity. Obesity is linked to cancers of the breast, colon, gallbladder and uterus.

✔ Include more garlic and onion in your meals. The amyl sulfides found in garlic and onions have been identified as providing protection against cancer.

✔ Aim for 25 to 30 grams of fiber from sources like whole-grain foods, fruits, vegetables and dried beans. The protective effects of fiber are associated with eating fiber-rich foods and not with taking fiber supplements. A diet that's high in fiber and low in fat may protect you from colon and rectal cancer.

✔ Eat more vegetables from the cabbage family (broccoli, cauliflower, brussels sprouts and kale); they contain the potent phytochemical sulforaphane. These cruciferous vegetables have been connected to a lower incidence of colon cancer, cancer of the esophagus, oral and pharyngeal cancers, breast cancer and thyroid cancer.

✔ Drink a cup of brewed tea daily. Catechins and polyphenols in tea are powerful antioxidants.

✔ Seek out selenium-rich foods. Selenium is found in seafood, meats, garlic and whole grains.

✔ A liberal macrobiotic eating style (a diet that includes whole grains, fish, nuts, seeds, tofu and vegetables) is consistent with dietary recommendations for preventing cancer.

✔ People who already have cancer should avoid macrobiotic diets of any kind, because they may not provide enough calories and protein to protect against the wasting associated with the disease.

✔ Avoid foods grilled at very high temperatures or crisply blackened, especially fatty foods. The smoke produced by the burning fat produces polycyclic aromatic hydrocarbons (PAHs) that can be carcinogenic. You can reduce the negative effects of grilling by trimming as much fat as possible from meats, by skinning poultry before broiling, and by not putting frozen meats on the grill.

✔ Reduce your consumption of smoked foods because they tend to absorb carcinogens that are similar chemically to the cigarette tars in tobacco smoke.

✔ Salt-cured, pickled and nitrite-cured foods (processed lunch meats and bacon) may increase the risk of cancer.

✔ If you drink alcohol, limit your intake to no more than 1 drink per day for women or 2 drinks per day for men. Excessive drinking increases your chances for liver cancer.

SUPPLEMENT SUGGESTIONS

▸ A multivitamin/mineral supplement with RDAs of 100 to 150 percent is recommended for those at risk for cancer or who have had cancer.

▸ There is mixed evidence on soy supplementation for those with cancer. At this time, supplements of soy isoflavones should be avoided.

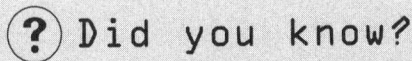

(?) Did you know?

Cancer takes its name from the crab-shaped stars in the constellation Cancer. When cells pile up, it's called a tumor. When they pile up into a fist- or ball-shape, which can be easily removed, they are usually benign. Malignant cancer cells tend to spread out more, like an open hand or the crab-shaped claws of the zodiac sign for the crab.

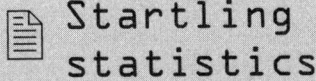

📄 Startling statistics

Medical research estimates that diet and nutrition factors can influence 70 percent of all preventable cancers and 35 percent of cancer deaths in the United States.

Cataracts

For most people, cataracts are a natural result of aging. In fact, cataracts are the leading cause of vision loss among adults aged 55 and older. Most people think of cataracts as a cloudy film that grows over the eyes, causing blurred or double vision. However, a cataract does not form on the eye, but rather within the eye. Although many people do develop cataracts in both eyes, cataracts will not spread from one eye to the other.

WHAT IS IT?

A cataract is a clouding of the eye lens that helps you focus light and produce clear, sharp images. The lens of each eye is contained in a sealed bag or capsule of fluid. As old cells die, they become trapped inside this capsule. Over time, cells accumulate, causing the lens to cloud, which makes images appear blurred or fuzzy. In the early stages, a cataract may not cause vision problems if the cloudiness affects only a small part of the lens. But over time, the cataract might grow larger and cloud more area, making it harder to see. Because less light can reach the retina through the clouding, vision becomes dull and blurry.

▶ Common symptoms

- ■ Cloudy vision

☞ Who's at risk?

- Those with a family history of cataracts
- Diabetics
- Alcoholics
- Those with a history of eye injuries
- Those with excessive exposure to sunlight
- Long-term steroid users

NUTRITION RECOMMENDATIONS

We're still in the beginning stages of learning which specific food components offer the best weapon to battle oxidation in the eye. One thing is certain: People who eat the most fruits and vegetables have the lowest rates of cataracts.

✔ *Eat plenty of fruits and vegetables. Aim for a minimum of five to nine servings each day.*

✔ *Add blueberries to cereals, pancakes, yogurt or just about anything. They are especially high in flavonoids that can help prevent eye damage.*

✔ *If you have diabetes, keep your blood sugar in tight control. Fluctuating blood sugar levels can damage the lens of the eye.*

✔ *Use fruit juices in place of water for cake mixes and muffin recipes.*

✔ *Add tomato or vegetable juice to soups and stews.*

SUPPLEMENT SUGGESTIONS

▸ Take a multivitamin/mineral supplement that provides 100 to 150 percent of the antioxidant nutrients vitamins C, E and beta-carotene daily.

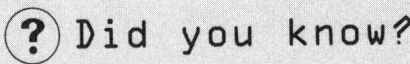

Did you know?

Much of the oxidation that happens to your eyes is the result of exposure to UV radiation from sunlight.

Wear a wide-brimmed hat and UVA and UVB protection sunglasses. Eye protection is especially critical between the hours of 10 a.m. and 4 p.m. Don't forget to include your children because UVA and UVB light damage is cumulative.

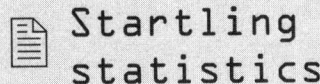

Startling statistics

Removal of cataracts is the most common surgery for Americans over the age of 65.

Ninety percent of people over age 75 have some type of cataract.

Depression

Of course, we all feel a little sad, dejected or blue now and then. Fleeting unhappiness may briefly cloud your horizon after you lose a job, break up with your lover or move to a new town. The profound mourning following the death of a loved one may last for several months—a completely normal response to a deeply felt emotional loss.

WHAT IS IT?

The key difference between sad feelings and a true major depression is that sad feelings eventually pass and depression does not. Depression is a serious disorder and should not be self-treated. If you experience the common symptoms of depression, seek the advice of a mental healthcare professional for diagnosis and treatment options.

☞ Who's at risk?

- Those with a family history of depression
- Those with lack of social support
- Those with a current or past history of alcohol or drug abuse
- Women aged 25 to 44
- Women who have just had a baby

NUTRITION RECOMMENDATIONS

✔ *Choose more complex carbohydrate foods to help boost serotonin levels. For example, choose a bagel instead of a donut.*

✔ *Avoid lots of processed foods and foods that are high in sugar.*

✔ *Avoid eating high-protein foods alone as snacks; they can lower tryptophan and serotonin levels in your brain.*

SUPPLEMENT SUGGESTIONS

▶ A multivitamin/mineral supplement with 100 to 150 percent of the RDA is recommended for those with, or at risk for, depression.

▶ Common symptoms

- Persistent sadness
- Fatigue
- Changes in appetite
- Loss of interest in ordinary activities
- Feelings of hopelessness
- Thoughts of suicide or self-harm

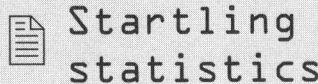

Startling statistics

Suicide is now the second leading cause of death among children and adolescents.

More than 80 percent of those treated with antidepressant medications respond favorably.

Diabetes

Diabetes is the fastest growing chronic disease in the United States. Diabetes cannot be cured yet, but it can be controlled. Sixteen million Americans have diabetes, which is a leading cause of blindness, foot and leg amputations, advanced kidney disease, and is a major contributor to heart attacks and strokes. Uncontrolled diabetes can complicate pregnancy, and birth defects are more common in babies born to women with diabetes. During the last 20 years, more people have died from diabetes than in all of the wars throughout the world in the last century.

WHAT IS IT?

Diabetes mellitus occurs when your body either cannot produce enough insulin or cannot properly use the insulin it does produce. If your pancreas doesn't make enough insulin or your body can't use insulin effectively, sugar (or glucose) will accumulate in your blood and spill into the urine.

There are three main types of diabetes.

• *Type 1 Diabetes:* thought to be an autoimmune disease in which the immune system attacks the insulin-producing beta cells in the pancreas and destroys them. The result is that the pancreas makes little or no insulin. Scientists do not know exactly what causes Type 1, but they believe that both genetic factors and viruses are involved.

• *Type 2 Diabetes:* the most common form of diabetes, accounting for 90 to 95 percent of all cases. It usually develops in adults over the age of 40, but is becoming more common in obese teens. In Type 2, the pancreas usually produces insulin, but the body cannot use it effectively.

• *Gestational Diabetes:* shows up only during pregnancy. This type usually disappears when the pregnancy is over, but women who have gestational diabetes have a greater risk of developing Type 2 diabetes. Older and obese women have the highest risk for gestational diabetes. Children born to mothers with gestational diabetes tend to have higher risk rates for other chronic diseases later in life.

▶ Common symptoms

- ■ Excessive thirst
- ■ Frequent urination
- ■ Weight loss
- ■ Fatigue or weakness
- ■ Frequent infections
- ■ Often, no symptoms are noticeable

☞ Who's at risk?

- • Those with a family history of diabetes
- • Women who have had gestational diabetes
- • Obese individuals
- • Inactive individuals
- • Native Americans

NUTRITION RECOMMENDATIONS

Maintaining a healthy weight is paramount when trying to prevent diabetes or slow down its progression. Excess body weight encourages insulin resistance, resulting in chronically high blood glucose. Losing as few as 5 to 10 pounds can bring blood glucose down and sometimes prevent the need for medication.

✔ *Find an eating plan that fits your lifestyle. Work with a dietitian to personalize how you eat to maximize glucose control and your enjoyment of food.*

✔ *Choose foods high in fiber, ideally 25 to 30 grams a day. Fiber slows digestion, which causes blood sugar to rise more slowly when you eat carbohydrates.*

✔ *Moderate exercise can help blunt the effects of the diabetes in people who already have it. For every 200 calories burned in physical activity, vigorous or not, insulin sensitivity increases by almost 2 percent. The higher the body's insulin sensitivity, the more effective insulin is at removing sugar from blood.*

✔ *Alcohol tends to lower blood sugar levels. If you consume alcohol you must carefully adjust your diet and medication. This should always be done with input from your physician or dietitian.*

✔ *Ideally, you should maintain a near-normal blood sugar level that is between 70 milligrams per deciliter (mg/dl) and 150 mg/dl. Frequently check blood sugar levels throughout the day. The Diabetes Control and Complication Trial, a 10-year nationwide study, demonstrated that by keeping blood sugar as close to normal as possible, people with Type 1 diabetes were able to reduce their risk of serious long-term complications by 50 percent or more.*

SUPPLEMENT SUGGESTIONS

▸ No alternative supplement or herbal aid can cure or treat diabetes. It can be life threatening to stop insulin, medication or your diet plan for false promises. Antioxidant vitamins may help mitigate the damaging effects of high blood glucose on cells, and reduce complications.

▸ A multivitamin/mineral supplement is recommended for all diabetics.

▸ There is evidence that some Type 2 diabetics may be deficient in chromium. Chromium helps insulin get glucose into the cells, so a shortage can mean higher blood sugar. Most Americans get about 50 micrograms of chromium a day from food; the recommended safe and adequate intake of chromium is 50 to 200 micrograms a day.

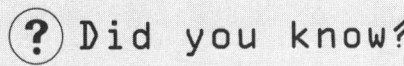

(?) Did you know?

For every two people with diagnosed diabetes, there's a third person who has the disease but doesn't know it. Because symptoms can be mild or nonexistent, many people realize they have it only when they develop one of its serious complications—blindness, nerve damage, kidney disease, heart disease or impotence.

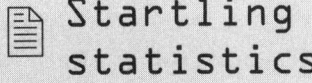

Startling statistics

The American Diabetes Association predicts a cure for some types of diabetes in the next decade. There are no cures today.

Epilepsy

Epileptic seizures are caused by electrical disturbances in the nerve cells in the brain. These seizures vary in their severity. Petit mal seizures are mild—the person will stare into space and may twitch slightly. Grand mal seizures are more extreme—the person will fall to the ground, become unconscious and have convulsions. Most seizures begin in childhood and just one-fourth of new epileptics are adults. Epilepsy, which stems from erratic surges in your brain's electrical rhythms, affects almost 2.5 million people.

Virtually everyone can have a seizure under the right circumstances. Each of us has a brain seizure threshold that makes us more or less resistant to seizures. Seizures can have many causes, including brain injury, poisoning, head trauma or stroke; these factors are not restricted to any age group, sex or race, and neither is epilepsy.

WHAT IS IT?

Epilepsy is sometimes called a seizure disorder, and is a chronic medical condition produced by temporary changes in the electrical function of the brain, causing seizures that affect awareness, movement or sensation. Infection, meningitis, rickets, malnutrition, hypoglycemia, head injuries, fever or allergies can cause epilepsy. Most of the time, the specific cause is not discovered for each person.

Long-term use of anticonvulsant medications is the most common treatment of epilepsy. As with any medication, the absorption of vitamins and minerals can be affected. Vitamin D, vitamin E vitamin B12 and folic acid are the nutrients most likely to be affected by long-term use of seizure-prevention drugs.

▶ Common symptoms

- Seizures

☞ Who's at risk?

People at risk for epilepsy include those who have or had:

- Brain injury during birth
- Brain injury from an accident
- Infectious brain or spinal cord disease
- History of seizures from high fever
- Toxic poisoning by lead, mercury, carbon monoxide and other agents
- Strokes

NUTRITION RECOMMENDATIONS

✔ Eat regularly timed meals and snack. If meals are missed or delayed, seizure frequency may increase.

✔ When used frequently or in large amounts, alcohol and caffeine may interfere with the anticonvulsant medication and may lower seizure threshold.

✔ All adults, and those children not on a specialized ketogenic diet, should choose a basic low-fat, nutrient-rich eating plan that includes plenty of fruits, vegetables and whole grains.

✔ *The ketogenic diet is sometimes used in young children who have not been successful at controlling seizures through medication. This diet is similar to metabolic starvation and is seldom successful in children over 16. The majority of calories allowed are from fatty foods. Children must be hospitalized to start the diet, and this way of eating is quite unpalatable and difficult to maintain.*

✔ *Ketogenic diets can be dangerous if not closely planned and monitored; do not attempt to try it on your own.*

SUPPLEMENT SUGGESTIONS

▶ A multivitamin/mineral supplement is recommended at 100 to 150 percent of the RDA for adults and children with epilepsy.

▶ A multivitamin/mineral supplement of 150 to 300 percent of the RDA for children following this specialized eating plan.

▶ Avoid extra folic acid supplements because they may decrease seizure control.

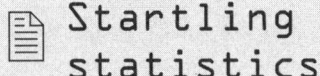

Startling statistics

Seizures and epilepsy will develop in 181,000 otherwise healthy Americans of all ages each year.

Children with epilepsy are at special risk for learning difficulties. Only 56 percent of people with epilepsy attended 4 years of high school, and 15 percent finished college, versus the national rates of 82 percent and 23 percent.

249

? Did you know?

Some evidence suggests that the sooner seizure disorders are diagnosed and the sooner effective treatment is started, the better the chances of a positive long-term outcome. Remission or longer seizure-free periods may be possible with prompt diagnosis and treatment and, when necessary, referral to an epilepsy center for specialized care.

Fibromyalgia

Fibromyalgia is not a new disease; it was described as early as the 1700s. In 1904, it was named fibrositis, and in the 1980s renamed fibromyalgia. Fibromyalgia syndrome (FMS) is not a form of arthritis because it does not affect the joints. It is instead a type of rheumatism of the soft tissues or muscles. FMS is also confused with chronic fatigue syndrome (CFS) because both involve generalized pain and have other symptoms that are similar.

Fibromyalgia is a common disorder affecting 5 million people in the United States and about 1.5 percent of the populations of other countries where it has been studied, such as Canada, Scandinavia, Germany, Italy and the Netherlands. It has also been recognized and studied in South Africa, Japan and Israel, and has been observed in India, Pakistan and Taiwan.

WHAT IS IT?

FMS is distinguished by chronic pain in the muscles, ligaments and tendons around joints. It is called a syndrome because it includes a set of conditions that always occur together. It now appears to be a disorder of the neuroendocrine system involving chemicals of the brain and blood that regulate how pain is perceived by the body.

▶ Common symptoms

- Gnawing, burning, shooting or radiating pain in the soft tissues
- Widespread aching that lasts more than three months
- Local tenderness at 11 of 18 specified sites
- Numbness and tingling in the arms and legs
- Muscle spasms and cramping, usually at night
- Fatigue
- Insomnia
- Severe tension headaches and migraines

☞ Who's at risk?

- Those with a family history of FMS
- Women aged 35 to 60

NUTRITION RECOMMENDATIONS

There is not enough information on potential links between fibromyalgia and diet to make many specific recommendations on food intake, other than to choose a healthful diet.

✔ *Increase fruits, vegetables and whole grains that are rich in antioxidant nutrients to help improve immune system.*

✔ *Cayenne from hot peppers stimulates blood flow, which may loosen up any blockages associated with stiff, inflamed joints.*

✔ *Aerobic exercise, such as swimming and walking, improves muscle fitness and reduces muscle pain and tenderness.*

SUPPLEMENT SUGGESTIONS

▶ As with most chronic diseases, a multivitamin/mineral supplement that provides 100 to 150 percent of the RDA is recommended.

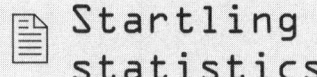
Startling statistics

FMS is actually more prevalent than rheumatoid arthritis, epilepsy or multiple sclerosis.

? Did you know?

In the past, many believed that FMS was just a psychological problem because it has no visible signs and could not be confirmed in laboratory tests. It is often misdiagnosed as arthritis or chronic fatigue syndrome, or diagnosis is delayed.

Gallstones

It's 2 a.m. and you're wide awake. Your stomach and chest are burning like those spicy cheese enchiladas you ate for dinner. Is it food poisoning? Was it that you ate too late? Then you remember this pain has been happening often lately. Maybe it's time to cut down on the late night fast food. Or could it possibly be something more … gallstones?

WHAT IS IT?

Gallstones are rock-like deposits of cholesterol (the same fat-like substance that clogs arteries), bilirubin and proteins that are found in the gallbladder (the pear-shaped organ located under the liver) or bile ducts. These stones can range in size from less than a pinhead to 3 inches across. The gallbladder stores and concentrates bile, a thick fluid that is produced by the liver, and releases it to aid in the digestion of fats.

▶ Common symptoms

- Feeling bloated and gassy, especially after eating fried or fatty foods
- Indigestion, nausea, vomiting
- Steady pain in the upper-right abdomen that lasts from 20 minutes to 5 hours
- Pain between the shoulder blades or in the right shoulder
- Severe abdominal pain with fever and sometimes yellow skin or eyes

☞ Who's at risk?

- Those with a family history of gallbladder disease
- Obese individuals
- People aged 50+
- Women taking estrogen
- Pregnant women
- Diabetics
- Those eating a low-fiber, high-fat diet

NUTRITION RECOMMENDATIONS

✔ *Maintain a healthy weight.*
✔ *Eat a diet high in fiber and low in refined carbohydrates, sugar and fat.*
✔ *Aim for 25 to 30 grams of dietary fiber each day.*
✔ *Eat a wide variety of fruits, vegetables and whole-grain foods.*
✔ *Choose breads and cereals with flax or psyllium added.*
✔ *Drink plenty of fluids, especially water.*

SUPPLEMENT SUGGESTIONS

▶ A multivitamin/mineral supplement with 100 to 150 percent of the RDA is recommend for people with gallstones.
▶ Consider 1 tablespoon of flaxseed or flaxseed oil daily; it may have some benefit in dissolving or reducing gallstones.

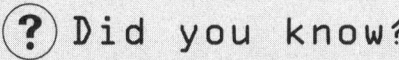

? Did you know?

While it may seem that the modern high-fat, fast-food diet is contributing to gallstones, the ailment is not a new phenomenon. Researchers have discovered a well-preserved Egyptian mummy from about 1500 B.C. with more than 30 intact gallstones.

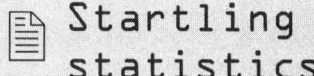

🖹 Startling statistics

More than 16 million Americans (most of them women) have gallstones.

Heartburn

The uncomfortable burning sensation you feel with heartburn has nothing to do with your heart. It's what you eat and when you eat it that causes the pain in your throat.

WHAT IS IT?

Heartburn is a backflow of acid from the stomach into the esophagus that causes the pain and discomfort. Just 1 to 2 teaspoons of this high-acid stomach solution can wreak havoc on the lining of your esophagus. Over time, this acid reflux can carve deep ulcers in your esophagus.

▶ Common symptoms

- ■ Burning sensation behind the breast bone
- ■ Gagging
- ■ Pain in throat or jaw

☞ Who's at risk?

- Pregnant women
- Obese individuals
- Fast eaters
- People who indulge in high-fat meals
- Smokers

NUTRITION RECOMMENDATIONS

✔ *Eat regular meals and snacks to prevent the buildup of stomach acid.*

✔ *Avoid fatty foods and fried foods.*

✔ *Avoid alcohol, chocolate and peppermint, especially in the evening, as they can cause the relaxation and opening of the esophagus.*

✔ *Avoid overeating or eating large meals.*

✔ *Don't eat or drink anything for three hours before you go to bed.*

✔ *Avoid tight clothing—especially at the waistline.*

SUPPLEMENT SUGGESTIONS

▶ If possible, avoid antacids, since they don't treat or prevent the underlying problem. Continued use of antacids can lead to permanent damage of the esophagus.

? Did you know?

If you sit up for at least 3 hours after meals, you may be able to prevent your heartburn.

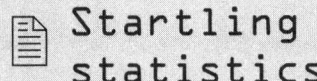

Startling statistics

In the United States, almost half of the population has heartburn at least once a month; 7 percent have it daily. Heartburn is even more common during pregnancy, with about 1 in 4 women reporting it daily at some point during their pregnancy.

Heart Disease

The most common first symptom of a heart attack may surprise you—it's death. That's right; sudden death is the first inkling that most people get signaling their heart trouble. If you have chest pains, shortness of breath or any of the other common symptoms, consider yourself fortunate.

WHAT IS IT?

Heart disease is our nation's second most common cause of death among both men and women of all racial and ethnic groups. At least 50 million Americans have some form of heart disease, including high blood pressure or high cholesterol. The American Heart Association estimates that the cost of heart disease in 1997 was $259 billion, including healthcare costs and lost productivity resulting from illness and death.

▶ Common symptoms

- Most individuals have no obvious symptoms of heart disease
- Shortness of breath
- Numbness or tingling sensations in arms
- Blue-tinged nail beds, which indicates lack of circulation
- Deep creases in earlobes

☞ Who's at risk?

- Those with a family history of heart disease
- Smokers
- Obese individuals
- Those who eat high-fat diets
- Individuals who avoid exercise

NUTRITION RECOMMENDATIONS

✔ Choose a low-fat eating plan that includes plenty of fruits, vegetables and whole grains.

✔ Trim all meat, poultry and fish of fatty deposits before cooking.

✔ Maintain a healthy weight, and get regular physical activity. Obesity is linked to most types of heart disease.

✔ Include more garlic and onion in your meals. The amyl sulfides found in garlic and onions have been identified as providing protection against heart disease.

✔ Substitute olive oil when possible in cooking; it is a healthier monounsaturated fat.

✔ Consider adding a 12-ounce glass of grape juice or one drink of red wine daily. Both may have a small benefit in reducing risk for heart disease.

✔ Aim for 25 to 30 grams of fiber from sources like whole-grain foods, fruits, vegetables and dried beans. The protective effects of fiber are associated with eating fiber-rich foods and not with taking fiber supplements. A diet that's high in fiber and low in fat may lower your risk of heart disease.

Supplement Suggestions

▶ A multivitamin/mineral supplement with 100 to 150 percent of the RDA is recommend for those with, or at risk for, heart disease.

▶ Consider vitamin E supplements that, when combined with your multivitamin, provide up to—but no more than—200 IU per day.

▶ Consider CoQ-10 supplements (see pages 176–177), but check with your healthcare provider for specific doses and to see if there may be interactions with any other medications you may take.

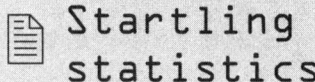
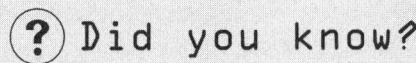

High Blood Pressure

We all have occasional high blood pressure. Temporary high blood pressure is a normal response to excitement, nervousness, physical exertion, anger, fatigue, coldness or smoking. Sustained high blood pressure is dangerous and affects nearly 60 million Americans, or one in four adults.

Historically, treatment of high blood pressure has alternated between an emphasis on diet and use of anti-hypertensive drugs. The use of drugs should never be the first option because of potential serious side effects. The nondrug approach is far more safe and effective.

High blood pressure is a significant risk factor for developing heart disease. Not only does hypertension increase the risk of heart attacks, but it also increases the risk of strokes and kidney disease. Of the 60 million people with hypertension, almost half are women.

WHAT IS IT?

Blood pressure is the measure of the force of blood against the walls of your arteries. A normal blood pressure for adults is 120/80. The first number (systolic) is the pressure when your heart is contracting. The second number (diastolic) is the pressure when your heart is relaxed. A blood pressure reading that is consistently more than 140/90 is considered hypertension.

▶ Common symptoms

- Headaches
- Fatigue
- Dizziness
- Heart palpitations
- Nosebleeds
- Blurred vision

But in many cases, no symptoms reveal themselves

☞ Who's at risk?

- Smokers
- Obese individuals
- African Americans
- Highly stressed individuals

Nutrition Recommendations

✔ Maintain a healthy weight. The benefits of weight loss can't be overemphasized. Overweight adults are 50 percent more likely to have hypertension than normal-weight adults.

✔ A modest weight loss of just 10 pounds, especially if you have lots of tummy fat, can often reduce elevated blood pressure to normal levels.

✔ Follow the Dietary Approaches to Stop Hypertension (DASH) diet: Eat 8 to 10 servings of fruits and vegetables each day; 2 to 3 servings of skim or low-fat dairy foods; 7 to 8 servings of grains; and up to 2 servings of lean meat daily. Also add 4 to 5 servings of nuts, seeds and beans over the course of a week.

✔ Drink less alcohol. Drinking three or more alcoholic beverages a day can raise blood pressure.

✔ Get regular exercise. It will help keep both your weight and blood pressure low.

✔ If eating less salt and fewer high-sodium foods helps lower your blood pressure, then stay on a low-sodium diet.

✔ Eating lots of fruits, vegetables and low-fat dairy products is more beneficial than cutting back on salt for most people.

✔ Foods rich in potassium, calcium and magnesium may help blunt the effects of sodium on your blood pressure.

✔ Try to eat at least one clove of garlic a day; it may have a small effect on lowering blood pressure. Add chopped garlic to stir-fry, sauces, salads and vegetables.

Supplement Suggestions

▸ CoQ-10 may help lower high blood pressure. Seek the advice of your healthcare provider for recommended dosage.

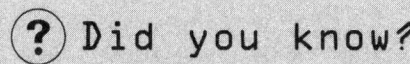
Did you know?

Uncontrolled high blood pressure increases loss of brain cells associated with aging. Fewer brain cells means your memory won't be as good and your thinking patterns will be fuzzier.

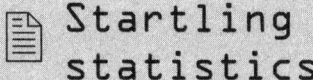
Startling statistics

Only about 10 percent of Americans with high blood pressure can lower blood pressure significantly with a low-sodium diet.

High Cholesterol

Your total cholesterol level includes different types of cholesterol in your blood. Actually, your total cholesterol is not as important as the ratio between the good and bad forms. High-density lipoproteins (HDL) are the good guys, and low-density lipoproteins (LDL) are the bad guys.

Your HDL level is a key factor in your risk for heart attack. For example, if your HDL level is low (below 35), you are at risk even if your total cholesterol is only 200. But if your HDL level is up (above 80), your risk is lower—even with total cholesterol as high as 240. The higher your HDL level, the better. LDL cholesterol is the bad stuff that clogs your arteries. You want low levels of the low-density lipoproteins. LDLs can be small or large; small LDLs have recently been linked to undesirable low levels of HDL and to high levels of triglycerides.

WHAT IS IT?

Cholesterol is a fat-like substance, and it is a building block of cells, vitamins and hormones in the body. Cholesterol is so essential that your liver manufactures all you need (up to 2000 mg/day). The standard definition of high cholesterol is having an excess of cholesterol in the blood, usually more than 200 mg/dl, although many doctors now use 180 mg/dl as the desirable maximum blood level.

▶ Common symptoms

■ No obvious symptoms
■ High cholesterol is usually found in the blood values on an annual checkup

☞ Who's at risk?

• Those with a family history of high cholesterol
• Those with poor eating habits (high saturated fat, processed foods, low fruit and vegetable consumption)
• People with a sedentary lifestyle
• Smokers
• Alcohol abusers

Nutrition Recommendations

In general:

✔ *Maintain a healthy weight.*

✔ *Eat more fruits and vegetables and a variety of whole grain breads and cereals.*

✔ *Choose lean meats, poultry and plenty of fish.*

✔ *Use skim or low-fat dairy products.*

✔ *Foods that have specific ability to dissolve blood fats and can therefore help reduce high cholesterol include: garlic, wheat germ, liquid chlorophyll, alfalfa sprouts, buckwheat, watercress, rice polishings, apples, celery and cherries.*

✔ *Consume foods high in water-soluble fiber: flaxseed, pectin, guar gum, oat bran onions, beans, legumes, soy and ginger.*

When dining out:

✔ *If you order a menu item that includes a heavy sauce, order the sauce on the side.*

✔ *Order grilled fish instead of red meat.*

✔ *Substitute a side of fresh fruit or vegetables instead of chips or French fries.*

When cooking:

✔ *Make broth-based soups instead of cream-based.*

✔ *Use olive oil in place of vegetable- or animal-based fats. Substitute applesauce, soft tofu or prune puree for oils in recipes.*

✔ *Buy trans-fat free (no hydrogenated oil) margarines.*

Supplement Suggestions

▶ Take a multivitamin/mineral supplement with 100 percent of the RDA. Extra B6 and folic acid may help if you have elevated homocysteine levels.

▶ Vitamin E (d-alpha-tocopherol "natural" form is recommended).

▶ Fish oil supplements may have the potential for lowering the risk for blocked blood vessels and heart attacks, but their current effectiveness and proper dosage haven't been determined.

▶ Coenzyme Q10 (CoQ-10) has potential as an antioxidant and could protect against heart disease. Because research into CoQ-10 is still at a relatively early stage, the use of supplements isn't advisable.

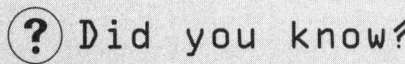

(?) Did you know?

Your LDL Levels

High	160 or above
Borderline high	130 to 159
Desirable	Below 130
Desirable for people with heart disease	Below 100

Your HDL Levels

Low	Below 35
Borderline low	35 to 39
Desirable	60 or more

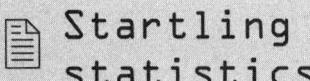

Startling statistics

At least 50 million Americans have some form of heart disease, including high blood pressure or high cholesterol. The American Heart Association estimates that the cost of heart disease in 1997 was $259 billion, including healthcare costs and lost productivity resulting from illness and death.

HIV/AIDS

What you eat is especially important when taking drug therapy for human immunodeficiency virus (HIV) infection. In many instances it can be the difference between success and failure with these medications. Malnutrition is a very serious problem for people with acquired immunodeficiency syndrome (AIDS). Life expectancy is directly related to how much body mass you can keep. Another source of malnutrition comes from ongoing infections, which change how nutrients are metabolized.

Food safety is as critical as good nutrition in the management of AIDS. Suppressed immunity dramatically increases the risk of food-borne disease and the severity of complications. There are bacteria and germs in almost everything we eat or drink. When levels of these contaminants get high enough, they can make you sick. It takes far less contamination to make you ill when you have AIDS.

WHAT IS IT?

Acquired immunodeficiency syndrome (AIDS) is a viral infection that causes a harmful antibody response in your immune system. The HIV (human immunodeficiency virus) gene actually gets into your cells and multiplies. As the HIV spreads, it weakens your immune system so that you are unable to fight off many normal infections. In a healthy immune system, the white blood cells surround a virus and destroy it. With AIDS, the HIV virus is surrounded but the white cells can't kill it, and the virus reproduces unchecked.

▶ **Common symptoms**

- Diarrhea
- Fatigue
- Fever
- Headaches
- Loss of appetite
- Swollen glands
- Thrush (white patches in the mouth)
- Weight loss

☞ **Who's at risk?**

- Those with multiple sex partners
- Those who have unprotected sex
- IV drug users
- Those with exposure to contaminated blood products or needles
- Children born to HIV-infected mother

NUTRITION RECOMMENDATIONS

Consult a registered dietitian as soon as diagnosed for a complete nutritional assessment including weight, height, body fat, lean muscle mass and body mass index (BMI). Keep as much lean body mass as possible by staying active and eating a variety of foods.

✔ *Focus on maintaining weight. Eating small, frequent meals can help increase the number of calories you can eat.*

✔ *Eat plenty of protein foods and antioxidant-rich fruits, vegetables and grains to keep your immune system strong.*

✔ *Thoroughly rinse all fruits and vegetables to avoid food-borne infections. Wash the outside of all fruits including melons, bananas and fruits not normally peeled.*

✔ *Never eat raw or undercooked eggs, soft ripe cheeses or ground meats unless they are well done. Use a food thermometer to check temperatures.*

✔ *Buy irradiated meats whenever possible.*

✔ *Drink bottled water or boil water before drinking.*

✔ *Try to decrease caffeine to help prevent stomach irritation.*

SUPPLEMENT SUGGESTIONS

▸ A multivitamin/mineral supplement that provides 100 to 150 percent of the RDA is recommended for those with HIV.

▸ If you are on antifolate drug treatment, you may need extra folic acid. Check with your healthcare provider.

▸ If you develop steatorrhea (fatty diarrhea), additional supplements of vitamins A, D, E and K are recommended.

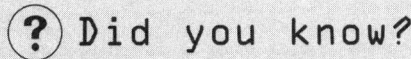

Did you know?

Use bleach or an antibacterial solution (1 tablespoon to 1 gallon water) to wipe kitchen surfaces. This is the most effective way to prevent the spread of food-borne disease.

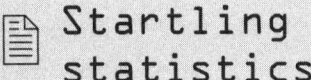

Startling statistics

A loss of 55 percent of lean muscle weight is practically a death sentence to those with AIDS.

Inflammatory Bowel Disease (IBD)

Crohn's disease and colitis are both types of inflammatory bowel disease (IBD). They are chronic diseases without a known cause or cure. An estimated 2 million Americans have been diagnosed with IBD. Malnutrition is a significant problem in IBD for several reasons. First, it's pretty miserable to live in chronic pain, which lowers the desire to eat. Second, scar tissue forms along the digestive tract as a result of inflammation. This scarring interferes with normal absorption of nutrients and decreases availability of nutrients and energy to your body. This is especially important in children when energy and high levels of nutrients are needed for growth.

WHAT IS IT?

Colitis is an inflammation of the inner lining of the digestive tract, affecting the colon or the rectum. Crohn's disease is an inflammation of all the layers of the digestive tract affecting any part from the mouth to the anus. It's because the symptoms and complications are similar that they both are grouped under the heading of IBD.

▶ **Common symptoms**

- Abdominal pain
- Cracks and abnormal openings connecting the bowel to the skin surface near the rectum
- Diarrhea
- Fever
- Skin that looks like hemorrhoids
- Sores in the anal area
- Weight loss

☞ **Who's at risk?**

- Those with a family history of these types of disorders
- Ashkenazi Jews

NUTRITION RECOMMENDATIONS

Individualization is the key to optimal nutrition if you have IBD. What may work for one person may not work so well for another person. Consult with a registered dietitian for personalized nutrition recommendations.

✔ *Choose foods that are rich in nutrients whenever possible. You may need to avoid some higher fiber foods if they cause pain or complications of your symptoms.*

✔ *Spread meals out over the course of the day. Five smaller meals instead of three large ones may help decrease side effects.*

✔ *If a particular food seems to intensify your symptoms, eliminate it for several weeks and then slowly reintroduce it to see if it has any effect.*

✔ *Children with IBD should increase their calorie and protein intake by 150 percent of the daily recommended allowance for their specific ages and heights. Studies indicate that for children with IBD, nutritional support is as important as medication for achieving remission.*

SUPPLEMENT SUGGESTIONS

▸ Avoid supplemental vitamins and minerals unless your healthcare specialist has specifically prescribed them; they usually do more harm than good.

▸ When you can't eat, try substituting a liquid diet meal (Carnation Instant Breakfast, Ensure, or Boost, for example) to provide calories and a source of nutrients.

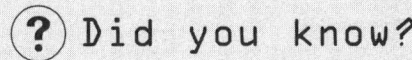

(?) Did you know?

IBD is one of the few conditions that benefits from a lower fiber intake. Too much roughage can irritate an already sensitive digestive tract.

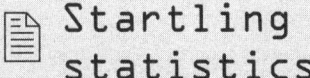

Startling statistics

People with ulcerative colitis face an increased risk of developing colon cancer, especially if the entire colon is involved and the disease exists for many years. It's important, therefore, to look for early signs that cancer may be developing. These precancerous changes, called dysplasia, may occur in the cells lining the colon.

Macular Degeneration

Macular degeneration is a leading cause of blindness in people over 55 years old. It can strike anyone and works slowly and silently to destroy your vision. Medical research studies show that as many as one-fourth of all persons over the age of 65 have a measurable level of macular degeneration. There is no treatment for this disease. The good news is that macular degeneration can be prevented or the progressive loss of sight slowed.

WHAT IS IT?

Macular degeneration is the deterioration and functional loss of the yellow spot on the retina that is responsible for central vision. The more the yellow spot deteriorates, the more vision is lost. Lutein is the yellow pigment that gives marigolds their golden yellow color. Zeaxanthin is another bright yellow pigment, which is almost identical in structure to lutein. Together, lutein and zeaxanthin are the pigments that color the tiny spot on your eye yellow. The density of yellow color is proportional to the amount of lutein and zeaxanthin it contains. Macular density gets worse as macular degeneration progresses because of the loss of these pigments.

▶ Common symptoms

- ■ Difficulty seeing fine print
- ■ Poor central vision
- ■ Difficulty seeing distant objects

☞ Who's at risk?

- People aged 50+

NUTRITION RECOMMENDATIONS

✔ Eat at least one or two servings daily of a dark green leafy vegetable such as spinach, kale or collard greens. These vegetables supply a high amount of lutein and zeaxanthin, the yellow carotenoid pigments necessary for the health of the macula.

✔ Eat a serving of blueberries every day. Blueberries are especially high in total antioxidative activity. Fresh or frozen blueberries are equally good choices.

✔ Eat a total of at least seven servings per day of vegetables or fruits with a high total antioxidant activity. By eating vegetables and fruits high in antioxidant activity, you can actually increase the total antioxidant activity of the blood.

✔ Drink a glass of red or purple grape juice or red wine every day for their protective antioxidant activity.

SUPPLEMENT SUGGESTIONS

▶ A multivitamin/mineral supplement with 100 to 150 percent of the RDA is recommended.

▶ Additional antioxidant supplements can be added to equal no more than 400 IU per day of vitamin E and 250 mg per day of vitamin C. Be sure to include the amounts of these nutrients in your multivitamin supplement before adding any extra to meet these totals.

? Did you know?

If you don't like blueberries, you can try bilberry extract (ranks even higher than blueberries for antioxidant capacity). However, eating whole fruit (blueberry or bilberry) may offer other beneficial substances that may not be present in the extract.

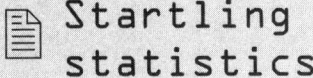 Startling statistics

Macular degeneration is the most common cause of legal blindness in the United States.

Menopause

Menopause, also referred to as "the change of life," is the point at which women stop ovulating. Menopause is not an ailment or disease, but a natural condition that occurs when the ovaries no longer produce enough estrogen to stimulate menstruation. The menopausal period affects each woman differently. For most women, menstrual cycles become less regular between ages 40 and 60.

WHAT IS IT?

Menopause results from the ovaries losing their ability to release hormones. The menopausal period can last up to five years, after which the cycles cease. Although estrogen levels drop during the post-menopausal period, the hormone does not completely disappear. Most of the symptoms associated with menopause may be the result of fluctuating estrogen levels.

▶ **Common symptoms**

- Depression
- Dizziness
- Headache
- Hot flashes
- Shortness of breath
- Weight gain

NUTRITION RECOMMENDATIONS

✔ *Maintain a healthy weight by increasing regular physical activity. Calorie needs decrease as your age increases. Since most women eat a minimal amount of calories to begin with, increasing caloric output is the best solution for preventing undesirable weight gain.*

✔ *Choose foods rich in calcium and magnesium to curb bone loss. It's still important to choose high-iron foods, since most women eat so few calories.*

✔ *Experiment with foods like soy and flaxseed to determine if they have a benefit in reducing your menopausal symptoms. Try just one at a time so that you can effectively judge its impact.*

SUPPLEMENT SUGGESTIONS

▶ If you can't or won't consume dairy products, choose a calcium carbonate or calcium citrate supplement.

▶ Less iron is required for menopausal women, because they no longer have monthly blood losses.

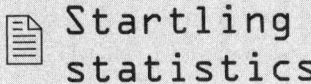

Migraine Headaches

It starts as a hot pain behind your eye and builds to a peak until you cannot stand light, noise or even the slightest touch. You just want to lie in dark silence. Migraine headaches are a whole dimension beyond headaches. Migraines tend to begin in your head, but as they progress, they can cause havoc on your whole body with severe head throbbing, nausea, vomiting, dizziness, cold hands, tremors and sensitivity to light and sound.

WHAT IS IT?

Electrical spasms in the back of the brain are thought to trigger migraines. These spasms cause blood vessels in the back part of the brain area to get smaller, while the vessels at the top of the brain widen. The inability of brain blood vessels to expand and contract at uniform rates causes throbbing pain and inflammation in the brain covering. When blood flow increases through larger vessels, the pressure on the smaller ones causes painful stretching as they try unsuccessfully to expand to allow for the heavier flow. Migraines can be temporary or can last a day or two.

Migraines are largely hereditary, and women tend to develop them three times more than men. Nearly 18 million Americans suffer migraines, and more than 157 million workdays are lost each year because of them, according to the National Headache Foundation in Chicago.

Many things can bring on an attack of migraine: changing hormone levels prior to menstruation or during ovulation, poor eating or sleeping habits, stress, chemicals in food (including additives and preservatives) or low blood sugar.

Magnesium may play a role in preventing or reducing the frequency of migraine headaches. Rich food sources of magnesium include cocoa, choco-late, most nuts, fish and shellfish, legumes, kelp, corn, soybean sprouts, lima beans, whole wheat muffins, taco shells, bran flakes, toasted wheat germ, brown rice, other grains and grain products, dried figs, dried pears, bananas and dark, leafy green vegetables. Feverfew is an herb that may also provide some relief from migraines.

Probably the best news for migraine sufferers is that chocolate has been taken off the list of foods that may trigger these severe headaches. Phenols in red wine and tyramine in aged cheese can increase hormone release that constricts blood vessels. When the vessels suddenly rebound to open, it causes a throbbing sensation. Caffeine can temporarily prevent a headache by dilating blood vessels, but too much will cause overdilation and that can be as painful as constriction. Some people are so sensitive to caffeine that even a little will cause a headache. Others get headaches from taking in too much. Food additives, including those containing sulfites, may cause headaches.

Another source of headaches is hunger. If pains occur right after you eat or drink a certain food, try eliminating that food.

▶ Common symptoms

- Pulsing or throbbing head pain
- Nausea
- Vomiting
- Extreme sensitivity to light or sound

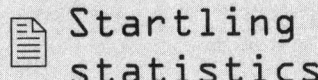
☞ Who's at risk?

• Those with a family history

NUTRITION RECOMMENDATIONS

There is no particular way of eating that universally impacts the occurrence of migraine headaches. If a particular food seems to trigger a reaction, avoid that food. Common triggers include red wine (phenols) and aged cheese (tyramine).

✔ *Include plenty of food sources of magnesium or consider a supplement if you can't regularly eat these foods.*

✔ *Smaller, more frequent meals may help prevent hunger, which can also be a headache trigger.*

SUPPLEMENT SUGGESTIONS

▶ A multivitamin/mineral supplement with 100 to 150 percent of the RDA is recommended for those prone to migraine headaches.

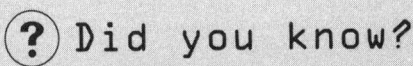
⑦ Did you know?

Alcohol tops the list of foods that affect the most people with migraines.

📄 Startling statistics

Some experts believe that individuals who have sensitive food triggers for migraines can eliminate up to 40 percent of their headaches simply by avoiding the offending foods.

Multiple Sclerosis (MS)

Nerve tracts in the brain and spinal cord are covered with a special coating called myelin. This coating acts as an insulating material and makes possible the speedy passage of electrical impulses from nerve to nerve. Myelin protects nerve fibers the same way that insulated cording protects electrical wires. In MS, the myelin becomes inflamed, swollen and detaches from the nerve fibers. Scar tissue can form in the gaps and slow or stop nerve impulses.

WHAT IS IT?

Multiple sclerosis (MS) is a progressive, degenerative disorder of the central nervous system. The disease is variable in its progression and affects various parts of the nervous system by destroying the myelin sheaths, which cover the nerves; this causes an inflammatory response. The symptoms include a staggering gait, blurred vision, dizziness, numbness, breathing difficulty, weakness, slurred speech, bladder and bowel problems, emotional problems and paralysis.

There is no known cure for MS, primarily because we're not sure what the causes may be. It is clear that both stress and malnutrition precede the onset of MS. A strong immune defense system to prevent infection is essential.

▶ Common symptoms

There is no typical MS. Most people with MS will experience more than one symptom, and though there are symptoms common to many people, no person would have all of them.

- Blurred vision
- Double vision
- Involuntary rapid eye movement
- Loss of balance
- Tremor
- Clumsiness of a limb
- Lack of coordination
- Spasms
- Burning feeling in an area of the body
- Slowing of speech
- Slurring of words
- Changes in rhythm of speech
- Difficulty in swallowing
- Fatigue
- Loss of bladder and or bowel control
- Impotence
- Short-term memory loss
- Difficulty concentrating

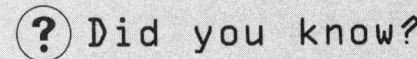
- Women
- People aged 10 to 59
- People in colder climates

NUTRITION RECOMMENDATIONS

While many different diets have been proposed as a treatment or even a cure for the signs and symptoms of MS, there is no evidence that any of them work.

✔ *The key to healthy eating is planning, especially when your energy is limited. Be realistic and determine menus that you are able to manage simply, especially when you are not feeling well.*

✔ *Make use of labor-saving storage devices such as lazy Susans and pegboards, and buy easy-to-open containers.*

✔ *Take advantage of precut fruits and vegetables, meats cut for stir-frys and other items that can save you time in the kitchen. These items may cost a little more, but they are worth it when your energy is low or you are in pain.*

✔ *Improve the nutritional value of convenience items by adding extra vegetables to packaged rice mixes and pasta sauce. Add extra tomatoes and fresh vegetables to pizza.*

✔ *Aim for at least two or three fish meals per week for their omega-3 fatty acid content.*

SUPPLEMENT SUGGESTIONS

▸ A general multivitamin and mineral supplement is recommended for those with MS. You may also want to consider a fish oil or flax oil supplement.

? Did you know?

MS appears to be a disease of temperate rather than tropical climates (i.e., there is more MS the farther one lives from the equator). In Northern Europe, particularly Scandinavia and Scotland, there is a high incidence of MS, which may reflect a specific susceptibility of the native population. A child moving from an equatorial to temperate area (or temperate to equatorial) before puberty acquires the risk of the area to which he/she has moved. The same relocation by an adolescent (or older person) retains the risk characteristic of the area from which he/she moved.

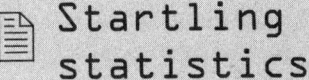

📄 Startling statistics

MS is not contagious or fatal. Most people with MS are employed and have a life span expectancy of 50 years or more after their initial diagnosis.

Osteoporosis

Osteoporosis (which literally means porous bones) is a bone-thinning disease affecting one out of every three postmenopausal women. Symptomless throughout most of life, osteoporosis usually first reveals itself as a hip or spine fracture in old age. While no cure exists for osteoporosis, its debilitating effects can be prevented.

The best protection against future bone loss is to build the best skeleton possible during the growth years of 9 to 19.

WHAT IS IT?

Bone is a living tissue, just like skin or muscle. Each year, 20 percent of bone tissue is replaced through a process called bone remodeling.

Two factors contribute to women's overall risk of osteoporosis: women's frame size and their hormones. Because women typically have smaller frames than men, they have less bone mass at adulthood than men and are thus more affected by any loss of bone. Testosterone protects men's bones as they age into their 60s and 70s. Women need estrogen for bone health and density; after menopause, estrogen levels fall.

Calcium aids in the bone-building process by helping increase bone density and strength. Infants have far more bone-building *osteoblasts* at work than bone-eating *osteoclasts*. That's why their milk-based diet is perfectly suited to provide so much calcium and vitamin D. During adolescence, bone development shifts into high gear. Nearly half of all bone is formed during the teen years. This is a time when calcium is crucial to building strong bones. Unfortunately, it is also a time when teens start replacing milk with soft drinks.

Bone health is perhaps the only health situation in which being overweight or obese most of your life is a positive. The heavier you are, the more stress you place on your bones, and that's a good thing. Weight-bearing exercise strengthens bone tissue. Of course, it's better for your overall health to have that extra weight in the form of dumbbells, not fat deposits on your body.

▶ Common symptoms

- None, most of the time
- Humpback
- Loss of height as you age

☞ Who's at risk?

- Older women
- Those who avoid dairy foods
- Those who had poor diets as children and teenagers
- Those who avoid weight-bearing exercise

NUTRITION RECOMMENDATIONS

✔ *Eat at least 1,000 to 1,500 mg of calcium per day from foods.*

✔ *Consume three calcium-rich dairy foods a day, along with generous amounts of green leafy vegetables. Choose* nondairy foods that have been fortified with extra calcium, such as orange juice and rice.

✔ Correct chronically low intakes of vitamin D, and possibly magnesium, boron, fluoride, vitamins K, B12, B6 and folic acid.

✔ Limit soft drinks because they are very high in phosphorus, which interferes with the ability to use calcium.

✔ Make regular weight-bearing exercise a part of your daily routine. Activities such as walking, jogging, bicycling and skiing all stress the long bones of the body against the pull of gravity, thus strengthening bone structure.

✔ Stop smoking. Smoking can be toxic to your bone cells and can reduce your body's absorption of calcium. Smokers tend to maintain a lean body weight, experience menopause earlier, and show an accelerated rate of postmenopausal bone loss.

✔ Limit alcohol intake. Alcohol is thought to reduce bone formation. Alcohol intoxication also increases the risk of accidents and falls.

✔ Consider hormone replacement therapy if you are past menopause. Estrogen therapy reduces bone reabsorption and retards or halts postmenopausal bone loss. Even when started as late as six years after menopause, estrogen prevents further loss of bone mass but does not restore it to premenopausal levels.

✔ Moderate your caffeine intake. Caffeine can increase urinary calcium excretion. Heavy intake of caffeine-containing beverages and foods along with poor calcium intake could compromise bone maintenance.

✔ Try kelp and other sea vegetables as condiments to flavor food such as soups, casseroles and salads. They are good sources of calcium, magnesium and trace minerals needed for strong and healthy bones.

✔ If you're lactose intolerant, try a chewable lactase supplement (like Lactaid or Dairy Ease) just before you eat dairy foods.

SUPPLEMENT SUGGESTIONS

▸ If you need to, use calcium supplements to assist in meeting your calcium needs, but remember that food sources are your best ally.

▸ Space calcium supplements for optimal absorption. Your body can best retain calcium in amounts of 500 mg or less. Figure out how many tablets (of 500 mg or less) you need to take through the day to get the recommended daily amount.

▸ Don't overdo calcium supplements. High calcium intake may interfere with magnesium absorption, which is also important in building bone tissue. Magnesium strengthens the matrix that helps bone act as a shock absorber.

(?) Did you know?

In the United States, the recommendations for daily calcium intake are twice as high as in other countries because Americans have greater urinary losses of calcium. Two theories suggest why this happens. First, typical American diets have a high ratio of phosphorus to calcium, about 5:1; the ideal ratio is 1:1. High levels of phosphorus reduce calcium absorption. Most soft drinks, particularly diet versions, are high in phosphorus, further upsetting the body's balance of phosphorus and calcium. Second, American diets tend to be high in protein. Protein foods are high in phosphorus and low in calcium, adding to the imbalance.

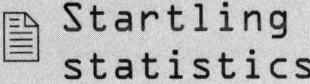 **Startling statistics**

Osteoporosis affects 25 million people in the United States, causes 1.5 million bone fractures a year, and costs $10 billion in medical costs annually.

Premenstrual Syndrome (PMS)

One factor that most women who suffer from PMS have in common is that they don't make smart food choices. PMS seems be one of those situations where marginal nutrient deficiencies add up to significant problems. Women who eat generous amount of nutrients from foods rarely suffer from symptoms of PMS, or have milder symptoms if they do experience PMS. Dietary supplements and herbs have been a popular area for intervention. PMS is a miserable experience and it's understandable that women will try almost anything to get relief.

WHAT IS IT?

PMS is not a disease in the classic sense. Women have reported more than 200 different symptoms in the days or weeks before their monthly menstrual periods. The most common symptoms include breast tenderness, abdominal bloating, weight gain, headaches, irritability and food cravings.

▶ Common symptoms

Symptoms vary greatly among women and include:

- Acne
- Anger
- Anxiety
- Backache
- Bloating
- Clumsiness
- Cramping
- Depression
- Food craving
- Headache
- Irritability
- Mood swings
- Muscle aches

☞ Who's at risk?

- Women with poor food intakes
- Those with a family history

NUTRITION RECOMMENDATIONS

✔ Get the nutrients you need from foods to compensate for the marginal deficiencies many women have that make them more prone to PMS.

✔ Break a sweat. Even moderate exercise can help reduce PMS symptoms. If you work up a sweat, the loss of water can help decrease bloating.

✔ If you crave sweets, opt for high-carbohydrate foods like potatoes, whole grain breads or crackers instead. They'll help soothe your mood without aggravating your PMS symptoms.

✔ Vitamin B6 is still sometimes prescribed in toxic doses by gynecologists and other healthcare providers for relief of premenstrual syndrome symptoms. Don't exceed more than 50 mg/day or you will be at risk for nerve damage.

✔ Limit consumption of alcohol, caffeine and salt if these compounds aggravate your symptoms. Alcohol may worsen mood swings and irritability. Caffeine can increase breast tenderness and nervousness. Foods high in sodium may increase bloating and fluid retention.

SUPPLEMENT SUGGESTIONS

▶ A multivitamin/mineral supplement of 100 to 150 percent of the RDA is recommended.

▶ High levels of B complex vitamins should be avoided.

▶ Consider fish oil supplements of 2 grams per day.

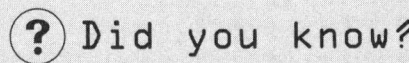

? Did you know?

In its most severe manifestation, women who suffer from PMS are unable to maintain jobs or relationships because of cyclical anger or similar symptoms. In some individuals, PMS is so severe that it causes suicidal and homicidal feelings.

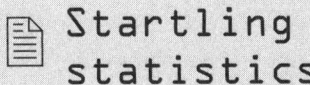

Startling statistics

There are 150 documented symptoms of PMS; however, most women normally report 30 to 40 multi-symptom complaints during any single cycle.

Ulcers

Milk and cream diets were once widely used in the treatment of ulcers, but the theory behind such treatment has since been abandoned. Currently, the main dietary rule is to eat regular, nutritious meals. Otherwise, use common sense and avoid foods that bother you.

WHAT IS IT?

A peptic ulcer is a sore or crater in the lining of the stomach or intestine that extends through the underlying layer of muscle. In the 1980s, extensive research proved that a bacteria—not excess stomach acid—was the cause for almost all ulcers. Stomach acid, other irritants and stress can all aggravate ulcer symptoms but they are not the cause. Alcohol, nicotine and tobacco cause the most acid production in the stomach. Other dietary factors may include tomatoes, citrus, spicy foods, chocolate and mint.

Calming down and taking it easy isn't good advice for the prevention of ulcers. It's a myth that anxiety, anger and type-A personalities cause ulcers. Recent research shows that the bacteria Helicobacter pylori cause most ulcers.

There are two main types of ulcers: duodenal and gastric. Duodenal ulcers are the more common variety and are located in the small intestine right next to the stomach. Gastric ulcers are true stomach ulcers that occur when stomach acid eats away at the stomach's lining. Esophageal ulcers are quite rare and are often a result of alcohol abuse.

▶ **Common symptoms**

- Abdominal pain
- Heartburn
- Nausea
- Vomiting
- Loss of appetite
- Bloating

☞ **Who's at risk?**

- People aged 70+
- Smokers
- Heavy alcohol users
- Those taking daily doses of aspirin or ibuprofen

Nutrition Recommendations

✔ *Ban bland diets. Since it's fairly clear that bacteria, not what you eat, causes most ulcers, there is no need to have a bland diet. There is no scientific evidence that a bland diet helps ulcers heal or reduces the painful symptoms that accompany ulcers.*

✔ *Don't overdose on iron supplements. Although people with bleeding ulcers can develop anemia and may need to take iron as a treatment, taking too much can irritate the stomach lining and thus the ulcer. Ask your doctor how much iron you need.*

✔ *Avoid foods that irritate your stomach. Use common sense: If it upsets your stomach when you eat it, don't. Everyone is different, but spicy foods (especially black pepper and chili powder) and fatty foods are common irritants.*

✔ *Stop smoking. Heavy smokers are more likely to develop duodenal ulcers than nonsmokers, largely because nicotine is thought to prevent the pancreas from secreting acid-neutralizing enzymes.*

✔ *Don't eat close to bedtime. Late-night eating stimulates the secretion of stomach acid while you sleep.*

✔ *Cut out alcohol. It irritates the lining of the digestive tract. If you must drink, dilute with water, soda or juice and eat food along with alcohol to help decrease its acid stimulating effect.*

Supplement Suggestions

▶ A multivitamin/mineral supplement with 100 to 150 percent of the RDA is recommended for those with ulcers.

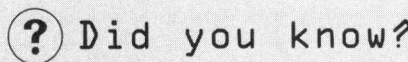

Did you know?

Spicy foods do not cause ulcers and drinking milk won't help them heal either. Today's recommendation is to eat what you like and avoid foods that disagree with you.

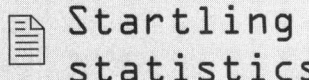

Startling statistics

Overzealous use of over-the-counter analgesics (such as aspirin, ibuprofen and naproxen), heavy alcohol use, and smoking exacerbate and may promote the development of ulcers.

Index

A

Acidophilus, 158–159
Adequate Intakes (AI), 20
Alcoholism, 226–227
    magnesium, 123
    nutrition recommendations,
        226
    pantothenic acid, 77
    riboflavin, 57
    risk for, 227
    supplement suggestions, 226
    symptoms, 226
    thiamin, 53
    ulcers, 279
    vitamin A, 34, 226
    vitamin B6, 65
    vitamin B12, 73
    vitamin E, 45
    zinc, 149
Alkalosis, 101
Allergies, food, 228–229
    facts and tips for, 229
    nutrition recommendations,
        229
    risk for, 229
    supplement suggestions, 229
    symptoms, 228
Alpha-lipoic acid (ALA), 160–161
Alzheimer's disease, 230–231
    facts and tips for, 231
    folic acid, 231
    nutrition recommendations,
        231
    potassium, 230
    risk for, 231
    selenium, 230
    supplement suggestions, 231
    symptoms, 230
    vitamin B12, 230
    zinc, 230
Amino acids, 13

Amino acids supplements, 15
Anaphylactic shock, 229
Anemia, iron deficiency, 120,
    127, 232–233
    facts and tips for, 233
    nutrition recommendations,
        232–233
    risk for, 232
    supplement suggestions, 233
    symptoms, 232
Antioxidants
    alpha-lipoic acid (ALA),
        160–161
    copper, 107
    flaxseed, 185
    introduction to, 15–16
    proanthocyanidins, 204–205
    quercetin, 210–211
    selenium, 141
    vitamin C, 37
    vitamin E, 45
    zinc, 149
Arginine, 162–163
Arthritis, osteo, 234–235
    boron, 95
    facts and tips for, 235
    glucosamine, 190–191, 235
    nutrition recommendations,
        234–235
    risk for, 234
    SAM-e, 214
    supplement suggestions, 235
    symptoms, 234
Arthritis, rheumatoid, 236 237
    facts and tips for, 237
    fiber, 237
    fish oil, 237
    flaxseed, 237
    nutrition recommendations,
        237
    omega-3 fatty acid, 237

    risk for, 236
    supplement suggestions, 237
    symptoms, 236
Asthma, 238–239
    beta-carotene, 238
    facts and tips for, 239
    nutrition recommendations,
        238
    risk for, 238
    selenium, 238
    supplement suggestions, 239
    symptoms, 238
    vitamin B6, 238, 239
    vitamin C, 238, 239
    vitamin E, 238

B

Bacteriocins, 206
Bad breath, 172
Bartter's syndrome, 101
Bee pollen, 164–165
Beriberi, 14
    thiamin, 53, 54
Beta-carotene, 168–169
    asthma, 238
    cataracts, 243
Biotin, 80–82
    deficiency of, 81
    facts and tips for, 81–82
    food sources of, 81
    metabolism, 81
    recommended intake of, 80
    skin and hair, 81
    toxicity levels of, 81
Blood clotting
    calcium, 97
    fish oils, 183
    flaxseed, 185
    spirulina, 221
    vitamin K, 48–49

Blood pressure, high, 258–259
  calcium, 259
  CoQ-10, 259
  facts and tips for, 259
  magnesium, 259
  nutrition recommendations, 259
  potassium, 259
  risk for, 258
  sodium, 144
  supplement suggestions, 259
  symptoms, 258
Bones and teeth
  boron, 94
  calcium, 97, 275
  copper, 107
  fluoride, 111
  magnesium, 123, 275
  manganese, 127
  phosphorus, 133
  vitamin A, 33
  vitamin D, 41
  vitamin K, 49
Boron, 94–95
  bones and teeth, 94
  deficiency of, 95
  facts and tips for, 95
  food sources of, 94
  hormonal balance, 94
  osteoarthritis, 95
  osteoporosis, 275
  recommended intake of, 94
  toxicity levels of, 95
Brain. See Nervous system and brain

C

Calcium, 96–99
  best supplements for, 99
  blood clotting, 97
  bones and teeth, 97, 275
  cardiovascular system, 97
  deficiency of, 98
  facts and tips for, 98–99
  food sources of, 97
  high blood pressure, 259
  menopause, 268

  nervous system and brain, 97
  osteoporosis, 275–276
  recommended intake of, 96
  soft drinks, 99, 275
  toxicity levels of, 98
  zinc, 149
Calories, need for, 12
Cancer, 240–241
  facts and tips for, 241
  fiber, 241
  fruits, 240–241
  nutrition recommendations, 240–241
  risk for, 240
  selenium, 241
  soy isoflavones, 241
  supplement suggestions, 241
  symptoms, 240
  vegetables, 240–241
  vitamin A, 33
Carbohydrates, 12–13
Cardiovascular system
  calcium, 97
  sodium, 144
Carnitine, 166–167
Carotenoids, 168–169
Cataracts, 242–243
  beta-carotene, 243
  facts and tips for, 243
  nutrition recommendations, 242
  risk for, 242
  supplement suggestions, 243
  symptoms, 242
  vitamin C, 243
  vitamin E, 243
Certified nutritional consultant (CNC), 27
Chitosan, 170–171
Chloride, 100–101
  deficiency of, 101
  fluid balance, 100
  food sources of, 100
  metabolism, 100
  nervous system and brain, 100
  recommended intake of, 100
  toxicity levels of, 101
Chlorophyll, 172–173

Cholesterol, high, 260–261
  cholestin, 174
  CoQ-10, 261
  facts and tips for, 261
  fish oil, 261
  folic acid, 261
  nutrition recommendations, 261
  risk for, 260
  supplement suggestions, 261
  symptoms, 260
  vitamin B6, 261
Cholestin, 174–175
Choline, 84–86
  deficiency of, 85
  facts and tips for, 85–86
  food sources of, 85
  function of, in body, 85
  lecithin, 84
  pregnancy, 85
  recommended intake of, 84
  toxicity levels of, 86
Chromium, 102–104
  deficiency of, 103
  diabetes, 247
  facts and tips for, 104
  food sources of, 103
  insulin, 103
  metabolism, 103
  recommended intake of, 102
  toxicity levels of, 104
Chromium piconolate, 104
Circulatory system
  magnesium, 123
  niacin, 61
  vitamin B6, 65
  vitamin B12, 73
  vitamin D, 41
  vitamin K, 49
Claims of dietary supplements
  health claims, 23
  nutrient-content claims, 23
  nutrition support claims, 23–24
  regulating, 24
  structure-function claims, 22
Cobalamin. See Vitamin B12
Cod liver, 183

Conditions
    alcoholism, 226–227
    allergies, food, 228–229
    Alzheimer's disease, 230–231
    anemia, iron deficiency, 232–233
    arthritis, osteo, 234–235
    arthritis, rheumatoid, 236–237
    asthma, 238–239
    cancer, 240–241
    cataracts, 242–243
    depression, 244–245
    diabetes, 246–247
    epilepsy, 248–249
    fibromyalgia, 250–251
    gallstones, 252–253
    heartburn, 254–255
    heart disease, 256–257
    high blood pressure, 258–259
    high cholesterol, 260–261
    HIV/AIDS, 262–263
    inflammatory bowel disease (IBD), 264–265
    macular degeneration, 266–267
    menopause, 268–269
    migraine headaches, 270–271
    multiple sclerosis, 272–273
    osteoporosis, 274–275
    premenstrual syndrome (PMS), 276–277
    ulcers, 278–279
Connective tissue
    vitamin C, 37
Copper, 106–108
    antioxidant action, 107
    bones and teeth, 107
    deficiency of, 107
    facts and tips for, 108
    food sources of, 107
    nervous system and brain, 107
    recommended intake of, 106, 108
    skin and hair, 107
    toxicity levels of, 107
    zinc, 107, 108
CoQ-10, 176–177
    heart disease, 257
    high blood pressure, 259
    high cholesterol, 261
Coumadin, 50
Creatine, 178–179
Cretinism, 115
Crohn's disease, 183

D

Daily Values (DVs), 20
Dehydroepiandrosterone (DHEA), 180–181
Depression, 244–245
    facts and tips for, 245
    nutrition recommendations, 244
    risk for, 244
    SAM-e, 214
    supplement suggestions, 244
    symptoms, 244
DHA, 182–183
Diabetes, 246–247
    chromium, 247
    facts and tips for, 247
    fiber, 247
    nutrition recommendations, 247
    risk for, 246
    supplement suggestions, 247
    symptoms, 246
    types of, 246
Dietary Reference Intakes (DRIs), 20
Digitalis, 98
Dilantin, 66, 98
DMAE , 85

E

Empty calories, 11
Energy production
    riboflavin, 57
Enzymes, 16
Eosinophilia-myalgia syndrome, 196
EPA, 182–183
Epilepsy, 248–249
    facts and tips for, 249
    folic acid, 249
    ketogenic diet, 249
    nutrition recommendations, 248–249
    risk for, 248
    supplement suggestions, 249
    symptoms, 248
Ergogenic aids, 16

F

Fast food, 11
Fat, dietary, 13
    Food Guide Pyramid, 17, 18
Fiber, 13
    arthritis, rheumatoid, 237
    cancer, 241
    diabetes, 247
    gallstones, 252
    heart disease, 256
Fibromyalgia, 250–251
    facts and tips for, 251
    nutrition recommendations, 251
    risk for, 250
    SAM-e, 214
    supplement suggestions, 251
    symptoms, 250
Fish oil, 182–183
    arthritis, rheumatoid, 237
    blood clotting, 183
    high cholesterol, 261
    premenstrual syndrome (PMS), 277
5-Hydroxytryptophan (5-HTP), 156–157
Flavonoids, 16, 210
Flaxseed, 184–185
    arthritis, rheumatoid, 237
    blood clotting, 185
    gallstones, 252
Fluid balance
    chloride, 100
    sodium, 144
Fluoride, 110–112
    bones and teeth, 111
    deficiency of, 111

facts and tips for, 112

food sources of, 111

mouth rinse, 111

osteoporosis, 275

recommended intake of, 110

toxicity levels of, 111

Folic acid, 68–70

  Alzheimer's disease, 231

  deficiency of, 69

  epilepsy, 249

  facts and tips for, 70

  food sources of, 69

  high cholesterol, 261

  immune system, 69

  metabolism, 69

  nervous system and brain, 69

  neural tube defects and, 23

  osteoporosis, 275

  pregnancy, 69

  recommended intake of, 68

  toxicity levels of, 70

Food Guide Pyramid, 16–18

  bread, cereal, rice and pasta, 17

  fats, oils and sweets, 17, 18

  fruits, 17, 18

  meat, poultry, fish, dry beans, eggs and nuts, 17, 18

  milk, yogurt and cheese, 17, 18

  vegetables, 17

Fructo-oligosaccharides (FOS), 186–187

Fruits

  cancer, 240–241

  Food Guide Pyramid, 17, 18

G

Gallstones, 252–253

  facts and tips for, 253

  fiber, 252

  flaxseed, 252

  nutrition recommendations, 252

  risk for, 252

  supplement suggestions, 252

  symptoms, 252

Gamma butyrolactone (GBL), 188–189

Glucosamine, 190–191

  osteoarthritis, 190–191, 235

Glucose tolerance factor (GTF), 103

Glycerol, 192–193

Goiter, 114, 115

H

Hair. *See* Skin and hair

Heartburn, 254–255

  facts and tips for, 255

  nutrition recommendations, 254

  risk for, 254

  supplement suggestions, 254

  symptoms, 254

Heart disease, 256–257

  CoQ-10, 257

  facts and tips for, 257

  fiber, 256

  nutrition recommendations, 256

  risk for, 256

  supplement suggestions, 257

  symptoms, 256

  vitamin D, 41

  vitamin E, 257

Hemochromatosis, 119

Herpes simplex, 162

High blood pressure. *See* Blood pressure, high

High cholesterol. *See* Cholesterol, high

HIV/AIDS, 262–263

  facts and tips for, 263

  nutrition recommendations, 263

  risk for, 262

  supplement suggestions, 263

  symptoms, 262

Hormonal balance

  boron, 94

  iodine, 115

  iron, 119

  manganese, 127

melatonin, 200–201

niacin, 61

pantothenic acid, 77

riboflavin, 57

role of, in body, 16

selenium, 141

vitamin C, 37

zinc, 149

Hypothyroidism, 115

I

Immune system

  enhancing with nutrition, 18–19

  folic acid, 69

  function of, 18–19

  iron, 119

  pantothenic acid, 77

  riboflavin, 57

  selenium, 141

  vitamin A, 33

  vitamin B12, 73

  vitamin C, 37

  vitamin E, 45

  zinc, 149

Inflammatory bowel disease (IBD), 264–265

  facts and tips for, 265

  nutrition recommendations, 265

  risk for, 264

  supplement suggestions, 265

  symptoms, 264

Inositol, 88–89

  facts and tips for, 89

  food sources of, 88

  function of, in body, 88

Insulin

  chromium, 103

Intrinsic factor, 73, 74

Iodine, 114–116

  deficiency of, 115

  facts and tips for, 116

  food sources of, 115

  hormonal balance, 115

  kelp, 194–195

  pregnancy, 115

recommended intake of, 114
toxicity levels of, 115
Iron, 118–121
    deficiency of, 120, 127,
        232–233
    facts and tips for, 120–121
    food sources of, 119
    hormonal balance, 119
    immune system, 119
    meat factor, 233
    metabolism, 119
    pregnancy, 118–119
    recommended intake of, 118
    tea and, 120, 121
    toxicity levels of, 120
    ulcers, 279
    vitamin C, 232–233
Isoflavones, 218–219

K

Kelp, 194–195
Keshan's disease, 141
Ketogenic diet, 249

L

Labels
    information required on, 23
Lactose intolerance, 16, 58, 275
Lecithin, 84, 198–199
Lignins, 184
Linoleic acid, 184
Lipoic acid, 160
L-tryptophan, 196–197
Lutein, 168–169
    macular degeneration, 266
Lycopene, 168–169

M

Macular degeneration, 266–267
    facts and tips for, 267
    lutein, 266
    nutrition recommendations,
        266
    risk for, 266
    supplement suggestions, 266

symptoms, 266
    vitamin C, 266
    vitamin E, 266
    zeaxanthin, 266
Magnesium, 122–124
    alcoholism, 123
    bones and teeth, 123, 275
    circulatory system, 123
    deficiency of, 124
    facts and tips for, 124
    food sources of, 123
    high blood pressure, 259
    menopause, 268
    metabolism, 123
    migraine headaches, 270–271
    recommended intake of, 122
    toxicity levels of, 124
Manganese, 126–128
    bones and teeth, 127
    deficiency of, 127
    facts and tips for, 127–128
    food sources of, 127
    hormonal balance, 127
    recommended intake of, 126
    toxicity levels of, 127
Measurements, for nutrients, 15
Meat factor, 233
Medical conditions. *See*
    Conditions
Melatonin, 200–201
Menkes disease, 107
Menopause, 268–269
    calcium, 268
    facts and tips for, 269
    magnesium, 268
    nutrition recommendations,
        268
    supplement suggestions, 268
    symptoms, 268
Metabolism
    biotin, 81
    chloride, 100
    chromium, 103
    differences in, and nutritional
        needs, 10
    folic acid, 69
    iron, 119
    magnesium, 123

pantothenic acid, 77
    phosphorus, 133
    potassium, 136
    vitamin B6, 65
    vitamin B12, 73
    zinc, 149
Migraine headaches, 270–271
    facts and tips for, 271
    magnesium, 270–271
    nutrition recommendations,
        271
    risk for, 271
    SAM-e, 214
    supplement suggestions, 271
    symptoms, 270
Minerals
    basic facts of, 19
    boron, 94–95
    calcium, 96–99
    chloride, 100–101
    chromium, 102–104
    colloidal, 14–15
    copper, 106–108
    defined, 14
    electrolytes, 14
    fluoride, 110–112
    heavy metals, 14
    introduction to, 14–15
    iodine, 114–116
    iron, 118–121
    magnesium, 122–124
    major minerals, 14
    manganese, 126–128
    molybdenum, 130–131
    nutrient recommended
        standards for, 20
    phosphorus, 132–134
    potassium, 136–138
    protecting your investment,
        25–26
    selenium, 140–142
    sodium, 144–146
    toxicity, 19, 21
    trace elements, 14
    type of claims allowed, 22–24
    zinc, 148–150
Molybdenum, 130–131
    deficiency of, 131

facts and tips for, 131
food sources of, 131
function of, in body, 131
recommended intake of, 130
Multiple sclerosis, 272–273
   facts and tips for, 273
   nutrition recommendations, 273
   omega-3 fatty acids, 273
   risk for, 273
   supplement suggestions, 273
   symptoms, 272

N

Nervous system and brain
   calcium, 97
   chloride, 100
   copper, 107
   folic acid, 69
   niacin, 61
   pantothenic acid, 77
   riboflavin, 57
   sodium, 144
   vitamin B6, 65
   vitamin B12, 73
   vitamin C, 37
   vitamin D, 41
Niacin, 13, 60–63
   circulation, 61
   deficiency of, 61
   facts and tips for, 62–63
   food sources of, 61
   hormonal balance, 61
   nervous system and brain, 61
   recommended intake of, 60
   toxicity levels of, 62
Night blindness
   vitamin A, 33
Nitrates, 37
Nutrition
   American diet and low consumption of nutrients, 10–11
   amino acids, 15
   antioxidants, 15–16
   calories, 12
   carbohydrates, 12–13

enzymes, 16
ergogenic aids, 16
expert evaluation of your, 26–27
fat, 13
fiber, 13
flavonoids, 16
Food Guide Pyramid, 16–18
hormones, 16
immune system and, 18–19
metabolism and nutritional needs, 10
minerals, 14–15
nutrient measures and conversions, 15
nutrient recommended standards for, 20
nutrition basics, 12
protein, 13
supplements' role in, 19
toxicity, 19, 21
vitamins, 13–14
water, 12
Nutritionist, 27

O

Omega-3 fatty acids, 182–183, 184
   arthritis, rheumatoid, 237
   multiple sclerosis (MS), 273
Osteoarthritis. *See* Arthritis, osteo
Osteomalacia, 98
Osteoporosis, 274–275
   boron, 275
   calcium, 275–276
   facts and tips for, 275
   fluoride, 275
   folic acid, 275
   nutrition recommendations, 274–275
   risk for, 274
   soft drinks, 274–275
   supplement suggestions, 275
   symptoms, 274
   vitamin B6, 275
   vitamin B12, 275

vitamin D, 275
vitamin K, 275

P

PABA, 202–203
Paget's disease, 111
Pantothenic acid, 76–78
   alcoholism, 77
   deficiency of, 77
   facts and tips for, 78
   food sources of, 77
   hormonal balance, 77
   immune system, 77
   metabolism, 77
   nervous system and brain, 77
   recommended intake of, 76
   toxicity levels of, 77
Pellagra, 60, 61, 62
Phosphorus, 132–134
   bones and teeth, 133
   deficiency of, 133
   facts and tips for, 134
   food sources of, 133
   metabolism, 133
   recommended intake of, 132
   soft drinks and, 132
   toxicity levels of, 133
Phytoestrogen, 218–219
Polycyclic aromatic hydrocarbons, 241
Potassium, 136–138
   Alzheimer's disease, 230
   deficiency of, 137
   facts and tips for, 138
   food sources of, 137
   high blood pressure, 259
   metabolism, 136
   recommended intake of, 136
   toxicity levels of, 137
Pregnancy
   choline, 85
   cod liver, 183
   folic acid, 23, 69
   iodine, 115
   iron, 118–119
   teratogenic toxicity, 21
   vitamin A, 34

vitamin C, 39
vitamin D, 42
zinc, 149
Premenstrual syndrome (PMS),
276–277
facts and tips for, 277
fish oil, 277
nutrition recommendations,
277
risk for, 276
supplement suggestions, 277
symptoms, 276
vitamin B6, 64–65, 277
Proanthocyanidins, 204–205
Probiotics, 186, 187, 206–207
Processed foods, 11
Protein, 13
Psyllium, 208–209
Pyridoxine. *See* Vitamin B6

Q

Quercetin, 210–211

R

Recommended Dietary
Allowances (RDAs), 20
Registered dietitian (RD), 26
Riboflavin, 13, 56–58
alcoholism, 57
deficiency of, 57
energy production, 57
facts and tips for, 58
food sources of, 57
hormonal balance, 57
immune system, 57
nervous system and brain, 57
recommended intake of, 56
toxicity levels of, 57
Rickets, 98
Royal jelly, 212–213

S

Salt Substitutes, 145
SAM-e, 214–215
Scurvy, 14, 38

Selenium, 140–142
Alzheimer's disease, 230
antioxidant action, 141
asthma, 238
cancer, 241
deficiency of, 142
facts and tips for, 142
food sources of, 141
hormonal balance, 141
immune system, 141
recommended intake of, 140
toxicity levels of, 142
Shark cartilage, 216–217
Skin and hair
biotin, 81
copper, 107
vitamin A, 33
zinc, 149
Sodium, 144–146
blood pressure, 144
cardiovascular system, 144
deficiency of, 145
facts and tips for, 146
fluid balance, 144
food sources of, 145
nervous system and brain, 144
recommended intake of, 144
salt substitutes, 145
toxicity levels of, 145
Soft drinks
calcium, 99, 275
osteoporosis, 274–275
Soy isoflavones, 218–219
cancer, 241
Spirulina, 220–221
Supplements
acidophilus, 158–159
alpha-lipoic acid (ALA),
160–161
arginine, 162–163
bee pollen, 164–165
carnitine, 166–167
carotenoids, 168–169
chitosan, 170–171
chlorophyll, 172–173
cholestin, 174–175
CoQ-10, 176–177
creatine, 178–179

dehydroepiandrosterone
(DHEA), 180–181
disintegration of, 22
dissolution of, 22
expiration of, 22
fish oils, 182–183
5-Hydroxytryptophan
(5-HTP), 156–157
flaxseed, 184–185
fructo-oligosaccharides (FOS),
186–187
gamma butyrolactone (GBL),
188–189
glucosamine, 190–191
glycerol, 192–193
inflated price of, 24
kelp, 194–195
labels and information
requirements, 23
lecithin, 198–199
list of ingredients for, 21
loose regulation of, 21
L-tryptophan, 196–197
melatonin, 200–201
PABA, 202–203
proanthocyanidins, 204–205
probiotics, 206–207
profits from, 24–25
protecting your investment,
25–26
psyllium, 208–209
purity of, 22
quality indicators for, 22
quercetin, 210–211
regulating claims of, 24
royal jelly, 212–213
SAM-e, 214–215
shark cartilage, 216–217
soy isoflavones, 218–219
spirulina, 220–221
strength of, 22
type of claims allowed, 22–24
USP standards, 21

T

Teeth. *See* Bones and teeth
Tetracycline, 98

Thiamin, 13, 52–54
    alcoholism, 53
    beriberi, 53
    deficiency of, 53
    facts and tips for, 54
    food sources of, 53
    recommended intake of, 52
    toxicity levels of, 54
Thioctic acid, 160
Tolerable Upper Intake Level
    (UL), 20
Toxicity
    acute or sudden, 19
    chronic, 19, 21
    teratogenic, 21
Tumor necrosis factor, 237

U

Ulcers, 278–279
    alcoholism, 279
    facts and tips for, 279
    iron, 279
    nutrition recommendations,
        279
    risk for, 278
    supplement suggestions, 279
    symptoms, 278
USP standards, 21

V

Vegetables
    cancer, 240–241
    Food Guide Pyramid, 17
Vision. *See also* Cataracts;
    Macular degeneration
    night blindness and vitamin A,
        33
    vitamin A, 33
Vitamins
    basic facts of, 19
    biotin, 80–82
    choline, 84–86
    defined, 14
    fat-soluble, 14
    folic acid, 68–70
    inflated price of, 24

inositol, 88–89
    introduction to, 13–14
    naming of, 13
    niacin, 60–63
    nutrient recommended
        standards for, 20
    pantothenic acid, 76–78
    profits from, 24–25
    protecting your investment,
        25–26
    riboflavin, 56–58
    synthetic vs. natural, 25
    thiamin, 52–54
    toxicity, 19, 21
    type of claims allowed, 22–24
    vitamin A, 32–35
    vitamin B6, 64–66
    vitamin B12, 72–74
    vitamin C, 36–39
    vitamin D, 40–42
    vitamin E, 44–46
    vitamin K, 48–50
    water-soluble, 14
Vitamin A, 32–35
    alcoholism, 34, 226
    bones and teeth, 33
    cancer, 33
    deficiency of, 33–34
    facts and tips for, 34
    as fat-soluble vitamin, 14
    food sources of, 33
    function of, in body, 33
    immune system, 33
    pregnancy, 34
    recommended intake of, 32
    skin and hair, 33
    toxicity levels of, 34
    vision, 33
Vitamin B1. *See* Thiamin
Vitamin B2. *See* Riboflavin
Vitamin B3. *See* Niacin
Vitamin B5. *See* Pantothenic acid
Vitamin B6, 64–66
    alcoholism, 65
    asthma, 238, 239
    circulatory system, 65
    deficiency of, 65
    facts and tips for, 66

food sources of, 65
    high cholesterol, 261
    metabolism, 65
    nervous system and brain, 64
    osteoporosis, 275
    premenstrual syndrome
        (PMS), 64–65, 277
    recommended intake of, 64
    toxicity levels of, 65
Vitamin B9. *See* Folic acid
Vitamin B12, 72–74
    alcoholism, 73
    Alzheimer's disease, 230
    circulatory system, 73
    facts and tips for, 74
    food sources of, 73–74
    immune system, 73
    metabolism, 73
    nervous system and brain, 73
    osteoporosis, 275
    recommended intake of, 72
    toxicity levels of, 74
Vitamin C, 36–39
    antioxidant action, 37
    asthma, 238, 239
    cataracts, 243
    connective tissue, 37
    deficiency of, 38
    facts and tips for, 39
    food sources of, 38
    hormonal balance, 37
    immune system, 37
    iron, 232–233
    macular degeneration, 266
    nervous system, 37
    pregnancy, 39
    recommended intake of, 36
    toxicity levels of, 38
    as water-soluble vitamin, 14
    wound healing, 38
Vitamin D, 40–42
    bones and teeth, 41
    deficiency of, 42
    facts and tips for, 42
    as fat-soluble vitamin, 14
    food sources of, 41
    heart and circulatory system,
        41

nervous system, 41
osteoporosis, 275
pregnancy, 42
recommended intake of, 40
toxicity levels of, 42
Vitamin E, 44–46
alcoholism, 45
antioxidant action, 45
asthma, 238
cataracts, 243
deficiency of, 45
facts and tips for, 46
as fat-soluble vitamin, 14
food sources of, 45
heart disease, 257
immune system, 45
macular degeneration, 266
recommended intake of, 44
synthetic vs. natural, 25
toxicity levels of, 45
Vitamin K, 48–50
blood clotting, 48–49
bones and teeth, 49
circulatory system, 49

deficiency of, 49
facts and tips for, 50
as fat-soluble vitamin, 14
food sources of, 49
newborns and, 50
osteoporosis, 275
recommended intake of, 48
toxicity levels of, 49

W

Water, 12
fluoride in, 111, 112
magnesium in, 124
Wernicke-Korsakoff syndrome, 227
Wilson's disease, 107, 131
Wound healing
vitamin C, 38

X

Xerophthalmia, 34

Z

Zeaxanthin, 168–169
macular degeneration, 266
Zinc, 148–150
alcoholism, 149
Alzheimer's disease, 230
antioxidant action, 149
calcium, 149
copper, 107, 108
deficiency of, 150
facts and tips for, 150
food sources of, 149–150
hormonal balance, 149
immune system, 149
metabolism, 149
pregnancy, 149
recommended intake of, 148
skin and hair, 149
toxicity levels of, 150

Recipes

Beef Brisket with Root Vegetables, 105
Black Bean, Corn & Green Chile Quesadillas, 139
Cannellini Bean, Chicken & Pesto Salad, 87
Chicken & Vegetables with Pasta, 59
Chicken Marinated in Yogurt with Lemon & Pepper, 67
Corn & Barley Salad, 109
Country-Style White Loaves, 83
Greek Lentil Salad, 71
Herb Garden Salad, 147
North African Tuna Kabobs, 43

Oven-Roasted Spuds, 125
Poached Salmon Steaks, 143
Pork Chops with Dried-Apple Stuffing, 55
Roast Leg of Lamb, 151
Sauteed Scallops, 117
Sesame Asparagus, 51
Shrimp Risotto with Lemon & Garlic, 47
Southwestern Hominy Soup, 79
Spring Fruit Crisp, 129
Swordfish Souvlaki, 135
Turkey Divan, 75
Wild Rice & Mushroom Soup, 113

fresh+healthy fresh+healthy fresh+healthy fresh+healthy

fresh+healthy fresh+healthy fresh+healthy fresh+healthy

fresh+healthy fresh+healthy fresh+healthy fresh+healthy

fresh+healthy fresh+healthy fresh+healthy fresh+healthy

fresh+healthy fresh+healthy fresh+healthy fresh+healthy

fresh+healthy fresh+healthy fresh+healthy fresh+healthy

fresh+healthy fresh+healthy fresh+healthy fresh+healthy

fresh+healthy fresh+healthy fresh+healthy fresh+healthy

fresh+healthy fresh+healthy fresh+healthy fresh+healthy

fresh+healthy fresh+healthy fresh+healthy fresh+healthy

fresh+healthy fresh+healthy fresh+healthy fresh+healthy

fresh+healthy fresh+healthy fresh+healthy fresh+healthy

fresh+healthy fresh+healthy fresh+healthy fresh+healthy

fresh+healthy fresh+healthy fresh+healthy fresh+healthy